Procalcitonin – Biochemistry and Clinical Diagnosis

UNI-MED

UNI-MED Verlag AG
Bremen - London - Boston

Priv.-Doz. Dr. med. habil. Michael Meisner
Städtisches Krankenhaus Dresden-Neustadt
Akademisches Lehrkrankenhaus der Technischen Universität Dresden
Industriestraße 40
01129 Dresden
Germany

Meisner, Michael:
Procalcitonin – Biochemistry and Clinical Diagnosis/Michael Meisner.-
1st edition – Bremen: UNI-MED, 2010
(UNI-MED SCIENCE)
ISBN 978-3-8374-1241-3
ISBN 978-1-84815-163-5

Printed in Europe

MEDICINE - STATE OF THE ART

UNI-MED Verlag AG, one of the leading medical publishing companies in Germany, presents its highly successful series of scientific textbooks, covering all medical subjects. The authors are specialists in their fields and present the topics precisely, comprehensively, and with the facility of quick reference in mind. The books will be most useful for all doctors who wish to keep up to date with the latest developments in medicine.

Preface and acknowledgements

Procalcitonin (PCT) is now measured in many hospitals as part of routine clinical diagnostic investigations. More than 10 years' practical experience and over 1500 publications on PCT allow a comprehensive assessment of the diagnostic possibilities and clinical application of this parameter.

PCT is currently undoubtedly the best "sepsis marker" that recognizes clinically relevant bacterial infections with a high degree of specificity and sensitivity – even in patients with immune system disorders and those on chemotherapy or immunosuppression.

In addition to indications and questions relating to the differential diagnosis that concern the assessment of the severity of a systemic inflammatory reaction and the prognosis associated with infection, information derived from the change of PCT over time is increasingly being incorporated into treatment decisions. This also allows questions on the need for, and efficacy or length of, antibiotic treatment to be answered.

This development is based both on the increasing experience with serial PCT measurements as well as the prognostic assessment of the success of treatment by means of the change in PCT. Furthermore, a series of intervention studies have established that an evaluation algorithm that integrates PCT and changes in it into treatment decisions facilitates the prescription of antibiotics individually tailored to the patient's needs. The question as to whether antibiotic treatment is necessary or not and when it can be stopped is determined on a more rational basis by the measurement of PCT than by a conventional approach.

Decisions based on PCT make possible a rigorous patient-tailored treatment regimen that must be examined on a daily basis and adapted based on other clinical information. This approach has many facets and, in order to be clinically successful, requires documentation of the causal or suspected focus for antibiotic prescription or corresponding interventions, accurate assessment of the nature of and risk from this focus (local and systemic risk, assessment of clinical importance, e.g. colonization or invasive infection), consideration of the immune response capability of the patient and the taking into account of current microbial isolates including the situation in relation to their resistance. The daily monitoring of the efficacy of treatment and the success of elimination of the infection focus is of special importance in order to determine when to end treatment at the correct time and on an individualized basis.

Furthermore, PCT allows risk assessment for the patient. Very low PCT levels are an indication that the risk of the patient suffering systemic complications from an infection or sepsis is rather unlikely, while if the levels are high or rising, mortality rates of over 20% have been described.

The patient's individual risk is information that may be used for the rapid and targeted application of the available treatment options in the affected patient or transfer of the patient to monitoring facilities. Patients at low risk can, in contrast, stay in facilities with less-intensive monitoring or be treated as outpatients.

Besides the highly specific infection and sepsis marker that procalcitonin is, it may in the future be helpful to measure other prognostic markers for risk assessment (e.g. for the assessment of the risk of organ dysfunction). In this way, treatment or monitoring individually tailored to the patient's needs can be undertaken, bearing in mind the available resources. In view of the limited resources of many health systems, the identification of at-risk patients is one possibility for improving treatment quality with comparatively low outlay.

At this point, I would like to thank the many scientists, doctors, colleagues and PhD students who are dealing with the topic of "sepsis" and procalcitonin and who are thus contributing to an ever-broader evidence base and better understanding of this disease and this parameter, including in relation to the clinical potential of the latter. I would also like to thank my family and my children for the patience that they have shown me in the production of this book.

I hope that it will act as an incentive to them and to others to keep working for continuing improvement in the medical treatment of critically ill patients.

Dresden, July 2010 *Michael Meisner*

Contents

1. Basic information 9

1.1. Procalcitonin, a marker protein for infection and sepsis . . . 9
1.2. Properties of PCT . . . 10
1.3. Diagnosis of severe bacterial infections and sepsis . . . 10
1.4. PCT and severity of disease . . . 10
1.5. Non-bacterial causes of elevated PCT levels . . . 12
1.6. Prognostic significance and evaluation of the progression of sepsis . . . 12
1.7. Influence on diagnostic and therapeutic decisions during the clinical visit . . . 14
1.8. Indication and monitoring of antibiotic therapy . . . 15
1.9. Stability and kinetics of PCT . . . 15
1.10. An overview of biochemical properties . . . 16

2. Primary indications 17

2.1. Diagnosis, progression evaluation, and therapy of bacterial infections and sepsis . . . 17
2.1.1. Diagnosis of sepsis, severe sepsis, and septic shock . . . 17
2.1.2. Differential diagnosis of severe bacterial infection and sepsis . . . 19
2.1.3. Evaluation of the severity of sepsis and the systemic inflammatory reaction . . . 22
2.1.4. Progression and prognostic significance . . . 23
2.1.5. Indication and control of antibiotic treatment . . . 25
2.2. PCT level measurement in specific clinical areas . . . 26
2.2.1. PCT in the intensive care unit . . . 26
2.2.2. PCT in the emergency room . . . 27
2.2.3. PCT in outpatient cases . . . 30

3. Biochemistry, pathophysiology 33

3.1. Procalcitonin (PCT), a soluble protein . . . 33
3.2. Genetics . . . 34
3.3. Mechanisms of induction and elimination of PCT . . . 35
3.4. Time behavior of induction and elimination . . . 36
3.5. Biological effects of PCT . . . 36

4. Laboratory chemistry 39

4.1. Methods of PCT level measurement . . . 39
4.2. Stability and half-life in vitro, preanalytical factors . . . 39
4.3. Normal values and reference ranges of PCT . . . 39

5. PCT as a marker of infection and sepsis: an evidence-based collection of data 40

5.1. Differential diagnosis of bacterial infections: SIRS and sepsis . . . 40
5.2. PCT as a marker of the progression of infection to sepsis, severe sepsis and septic shock . . . 45
5.3. Interpretation of PCT in the clinical context . . . 46
5.4. PCT: a marker of infection or of inflammation? . . . 46
5.5. Comparison with other markers . . . 48

6. Use of PCT for the control of antibiotic therapy **52**
6.1. Basics of an individual, patient-adapted antibiotic treatment using PCT.......52
6.2. PCT-controlled antibiotic therapy in airway infections.......57
6.2.1. Overview of current studies.......57
6.2.2. Patients with suspicion of infections of the upper airways in the emergency room: the "ProResp" study.......58
6.2.3. PCT, antibiotic therapy, and exacerbation of COPD: the "ProCOLD" study.......59
6.2.4. Outpatients with suspicion of airway infections: the "PARTI" study.......60
6.2.5. Individual, patient-adapted treatment of community-acquired pneumonia with PCT: the "ProCAP" study.......60
6.3. Control of antibiotic treatment in patients in intensive care with sepsis, severe sepsis and septic shock.......62

7. Use for special indications **65**
7.1. Diagnostic use of PCT in patients with pneumonia.......65
7.2. Bacteremia.......67
7.3. Bacterial endocarditis.......68
7.4. Acute bacterial meningitis.......69
7.5. Differential diagnosis of viral diseases.......71
7.6. Fungal diseases: Aspergillus and candida infections.......72
7.7. Autoimmune diseases.......73
7.8. Allergic diseases.......74
7.9. Pancreatitis.......74
7.10. Vesicourethral reflux, pyelonephritis, and urinary tract infections.......76

8. Exceptions and special cases **79**
8.1. PCT induction without indication of a bacterial focus.......79
8.2. Induction of PCT after surgical interventions and trauma.......81
8.3. PCT after organ transplantation.......85
8.4. PCT in renal insufficiency.......86
8.5. Tumor illnesses.......87
8.6. Hematological/oncological illnesses, chemotherapy.......88
8.7. PCT in patients with leukopenia.......90
8.8. Bone marrow transplantation and transplantation of hematopoetic stem cells.......91

9. Children and newborns **92**
9.1. Measuring PCT levels in children.......92
9.2. The first days after birth: diagnosing newborn sepsis.......93
9.3. Infants (>3 days), toddlers and children.......97

10. Frequently asked questions **103**

11. Literature **106**

Index **123**

1. Basic information

1.1. Procalcitonin, a marker protein for infection and sepsis

Procalcitonin (PCT) is a diagnostic marker of severe bacterial infection and sepsis. Clinical PCT level measurement has gained worldwide acceptance in the last 10 years. PCT is a functional protein consisting of 114 to 116 amino acids (☞ Figure 1.1). It is an immune modulator with various functions, and represents a "new" type of immunologically active protein, differentiating it from other groups of previously known inflammatorily active molecules, such as the cytokines, leukocytary surface markers, acute phase proteins, or clinically detectable signs of inflammation. Procalcitonin has special functions and the body regulates its levels very strictly. The protein thus has its own diagnostic profile. These specific properties are the reason the marker was introduced in routine diagnostics, since it provides interesting diagnostic information during clinical use.

PCT is a particularly good indicator of the presence of a bacterially induced systemic inflammatory reaction. Bacterial infections characterized by a systemic inflammatory reaction induce PCT, resulting in elevated levels in the plasma (PCT >0.1 ng/ml) (☞ Figure 1.2). At levels of 0.5 ng/ml, there is always a suspicion of sepsis, but usually (depending on the severity of the inflammatory reaction) sepsis produces even much higher levels. In severe sepsis or septic shock, frequently plasma concentrations of 2 to 10 ng/ml are seen and sometimes even higher values are measured. Although concentrations of more than 100 or even 1,000 ng/ml can occur in some patients, these cases are extremely rare. In local bacterial infections, elevated PCT levels can also be found in the plasma, if the inflammatory reaction has reached a certain extent. In such cases, concentrations usually are below 0.5 ng/ml, which is the threshold level cited for a diagnosis of sepsis. The normal range of PCT can be considered to be <0.1 ng/ml since over 95% of the levels of healthy subjects fall within this range (1). Starting at a threshold level of 0.5 ng/ml, sepsis or a systemic inflammatory reaction should always be considered if other causes cannot explain the elevated PCT levels.

PCT is primarily a measurement for the diagnosis of systemic inflammatory reactions triggered by bacterial infections.

Serum or plasma concentrations of soluble protein in healthy people are generally below 0.1 ng/ml (normal range). For levels of over 0.5 ng/ml, sepsis should be considered.

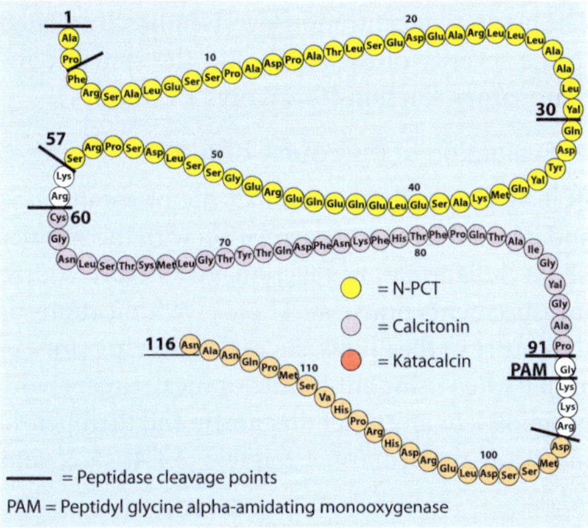

Figure 1.1: Schematic representation of PCT's amino acid sequence, its fragments, and possible peptidase cleavage points.

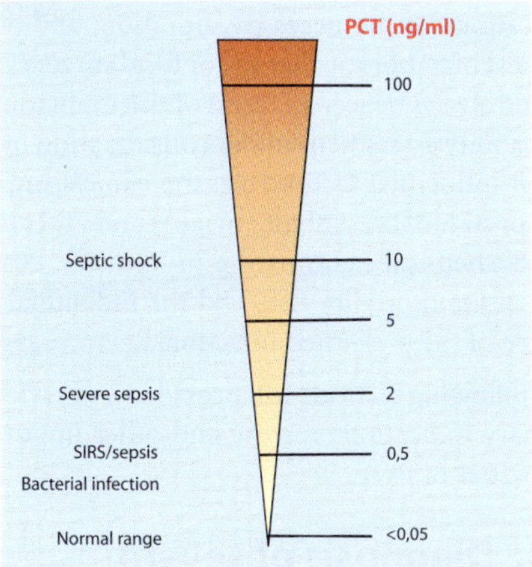

Figure 1.2: Serum or plasma concentrations of PCT are generally related to the degree of severity of "systemic inflammatory reactions" due to bacterial infection. It thus has an indirect relationship – taking into consideration any therapeutic procedures and idiosyncrasies – with the mortality risk of an illness.

1.2. Properties of PCT

The success of the diagnostic use of PCT in clinical practice is primarily based on the following properties and the resulting indications:

▶ Diagnosis of severe bacterial infection and sepsis

PCT has a relative specificity for inflammatory reactions triggered by bacterial infections (☞ Chapter 2.1., Figure 2.1).

▶ Evaluation of severity of sepsis

The plasma concentration level is indirectly related to the severity of the sepsis and the systemic inflammatory reaction (☞ Figures 1.2 and 1.4).

▶ Evaluation of the course of sepsis

PCT's plasma elimination half-life of about a day and its relatively good correlation with the severity of the inflammatory reaction make daily course measurements practical. These give indications of the course of the illness, success of therapy (for example when using antibiotics or focal surgery), the prognosis, or any other diagnostic and therapeutic measures needed (☞ Chapters 2.1.4., 5.2. and 6.1.).

▶ Indication and follow-up of antibiotic therapy

Since PCT levels are known to reflect the severity and course of infection, particularly bacterial infection, measured values can provide important indications of the necessity, duration, and effectiveness of antibiotic therapy or focal surgery. This should always be seen in terms of risk evaluation or probability assessment under consideration of different influential factors, e.g. the clinical impression or state of the patient, imaging and other laboratory chemical examination procedures, evaluation of the mortality risk, and the individual risk profile of the presumed infection.

The following sections will provide an overview of primary indications for use and other important properties of PCT.

1.3. Diagnosis of severe bacterial infections and sepsis

Bacterial infections induce PCT in measurable concentrations only after they have triggered an inflammatory response (local or systemic) and this response has reached a certain severity. That means that if PCT is increased, a systemic inflammatory reaction resulting from infection must be assumed (diagnosis of sepsis). Increased PCT levels indicate a possible risk for the patient (☞ Figures 1.2 and 1.4). Here, immediate therapy is generally needed. Simple local bacterial infections, on the other hand, may not always induce PCT. The conclusion that a PCT measurement can be used to exclude any type of bacterial infection is thus not a valid one, since local infections often induce very little PCT. For very low PCT levels, however, the risk of sepsis is low, and there is usually sufficient time to weigh the necessity of an antibiotic treatment against more thorough examination.

Even non-bacterial inflammatory conditions can induce PCT. However, PCT is generally induced more strongly by bacterial infections than by other inflammatory reactions (for some exceptions, ☞ Chapter 8. and following). This can be used to formulate a differential diagnosis. Viral infections, autoimmune diseases, transplant rejection, and allergic reactions generally induce no PCT. Even for cardiologically (hemodynamically) characterized arterial hypotension or perfusion abnormalities, e.g. pulmonary embolisms, cardiogenic shock, or low volume, very little or no PCT is initially induced. However, over the later course of the disease (e.g. for prolonged cardiogenic shock or if catecholamine administration is necessary), PCT levels may rise.

1.4. PCT and severity of disease

For the mortality risk of a sepsis, but also other intensive care illnesses, the degree of organ dysfunction is of paramount importance (☞ Figure 1.3). For example, mortality risk rises indirectly with the SOFA score (SOFA, Sequential Organ Failure Assessment (2)) but also with the severity of sepsis (see ACCP/SCCM_Criteria of Sepsis) (☞ Table 1.1). This applies both to patients upon admission to the hospital and also to the progression of the illness in the hospital (☞ Figure 1.3).

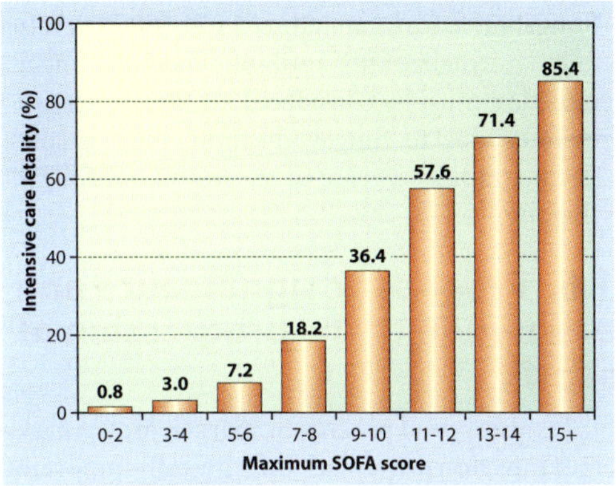

Figure 1.3: Mortality in German intensive care units depending on the increase in SOFA score in the hospital (difference between Day 1 and maximum). Columns: Mortality in percent; rows: case number. The model is based on data from 36 intensive care units, 45,000 patients, and 200,000 days of treatment during 2005. With the kind approval of C. Waydhas, DIVI).

PCT reflects this increased risk well, since PCT levels are related to the severity of systemic infection in sepsis, severe sepsis, or septic shock. PCT levels in the presence of organ dysfunction resulting from infection (diagnosed as "severe sepsis" or "septic shock") are generally markedly higher than in patients without organ dysfunction (☞ Figure 1.4 and 5.8). Thus PCT is also an indicator of mortality (370). This particularly applies to the evaluation of the course of PCT values (20, 36, 157).

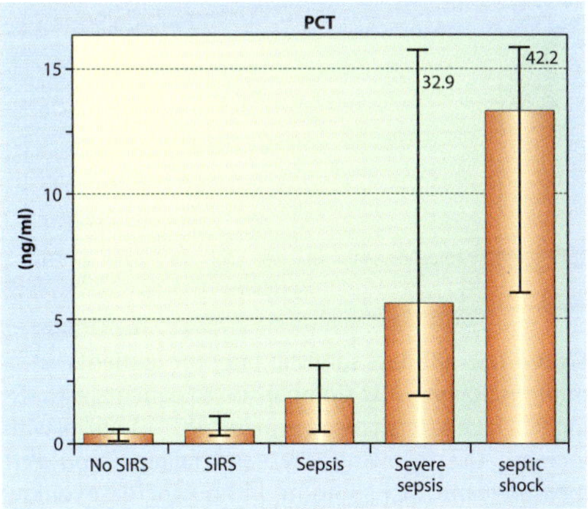

Figure 1.4: PCT levels for the diagnoses "Systemic Inflammatory Response Syndrome" (SIRS) (see ACCP/SCCM definitions of sepsis (5)), no sepsis, SIRS, sepsis, severe sepsis, and septic shock (6).

Increasing severity of sepsis also generally results in higher PCT levels. In "severe sepsis" or "septic shock" (sepsis with organ dysfunction), PCT is usually elevated significantly above the limit of 0.5 ng/ml (frequently above 2 ng/ml). Here, the patient is at risk of death. Therapeutic and diagnostic treatment is urgent.

Illness	Mortality (3) (1995)	Mortality (4) (2006)
No sepsis/SIRS	7% (SIRS)	14% ("no sepsis")
Sepsis	16%	27%
Severe sepsis	20%	32%
Septic shock	46%	54%

Table 1.1: Mortality of SIRS and sepsis (according to Rangel-Frausto, 1995 (3) and Vincent, 2006 (4)).

The degree of induction of PCT depends primarily on two factors:

- the severity of the inflammatory reaction ("sepsis, severe sepsis, septic shock")
- a bacterial infection as the cause of the illness

The good correlation with the severity of a sepsis is the basis for the FDA (Food and Drug Administration) approval of PCT as a marker of sepsis for clinical use in the United States.

The approval says, among other things: PCT is intended for use in conjunction with other laboratory findings and clinical assessments to aid in the risk assessment of critically ill patients on their first day of ICU admission for progression to severe sepsis and septic shock.

At present, the FDA approval lists, among others, the following interpretation rules:

*"**PCT >2 ng/ml:** These values on the first day of admission to intensive care indicate high risk for progression to severe sepsis or septic shock.*

***PCT <0.5 ng/ml:** These values do not exclude the possibility of infection, because locally limited infections (without systemic inflammatory reactions) may also be associated with these levels. If the PCT measurement is made very early (e.g. within 6 hours of onset of illness), the levels may also still be low.*

PCT 0.5-2 ng/ml: "PCT levels between 0.5 and 2 ng/ml should be evaluated carefully and the specific background and condition of each patient evaluated individually, since there are different non-infectious illnesses in which PCT can be induced."

The following sections include detailed information on individual indications, including references to clinical studies.

1.5. Non-bacterial causes of elevated PCT levels

PCT is a comparatively specific marker for severe bacterial infections or sepsis. However, individual situations are known in which – partly depending on the severity of the illness – PCT is still induced, without the presence of a bacterial infection (☞ Section 8.1). These are often severely traumatic events or situations in which – independent of any specific bacterial focus – an endotoxin burden is placed on the body, e.g. after significant abdominal procedures, abdominal trauma, severe generalized microcirculation problems with high catecholamine requirements, severe MODS, severe pancreatitis, or severe liver damage. If such situations arise, determinations of the course of the illness considering the individual situation may at least partly differentiate the "non-specific" (usually event-specific) PCT production from septically induced PCT. Medical knowledge and observation of the course of the illness increase diagnostic reliability in individual cases. If this fails, the PCT level cannot be interpreted or must be seen as a septically induced level in case of doubt.

Even severe fungal infections can induce PCT (☞ Section 7.6.). There are patients, however, in which no PCT is induced (7-9). In fungal infections, the expected PCT levels are often lower than for bacteremia. For example, candidiasis only seldom results in PCT levels of more than 5 ng/ml (10, 11). If PCT levels do not respond sufficiently to antibiotic therapy, this may be an indication of a fungal infection.

Fungal infections can induce PCT. If PCT levels fail to normalize after antibiotic therapy, fungal infection must be considered. If PCT levels are elevated due to fungal infection, they usually decline rapidly in case of successful antifungal therapy.

1.6. Prognostic significance and evaluation of the progression of sepsis

PCT is also a good prognostic marker. Many markers of infection largely lack this clinically important property (e.g. CRP, LBP, sTREM, endotoxins). Based on CRP, for example, it is nearly impossible to make any prognostic statements, since this protein correlates only poorly with the severity of the illness, and the kinetics of the plasma level are relatively slow. PCT, on the other hand, has shown prognostic properties in many studies, particularly when the progression of levels is considered in the interpretation (☞ Figures 1.5 and 5.2) (12, 16-21, 157).

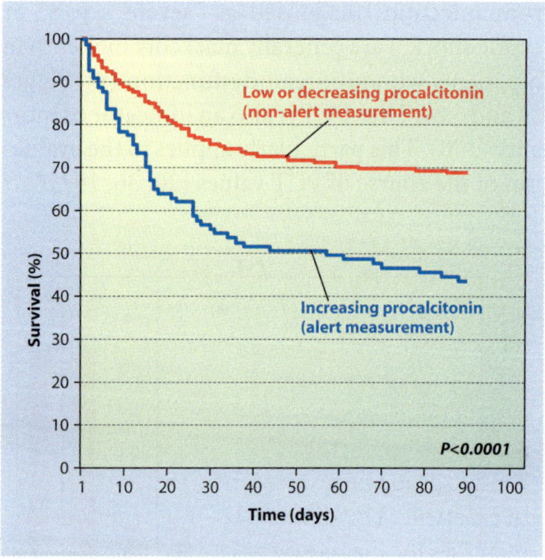

Figure 1.5: 90-day survival rate for patients in a multidisciplinary ICU. Comparison to patients with rising PCT levels (*"alert measurement"*, PCT ≥1 ng/ml with increase the following day), and falling (*"non-alert measurement"*, PCT ≥1 ng/ml without increase) or low PCT levels (PCT <1 ng/ml), respectively (n=472 patients) [157].

PCT has good prognostic properties, since the marker correlates with the severity of the illness and its progression over time (e.g. with the success of therapy).

Although the absolute level of PCT has no direct influence on the prognosis of the illness, very elevated or persistently elevated PCT levels are often a sign of severe illness with a high risk of organ dysfunction. Here, the mortality risk is usually significantly higher than for normal or only slightly elevated PCT values (☞ Figures 1.3 and 1.4) (157, 38, 12, 36). Early and successful treatment, however, can lead to a prognostically favorable progression in these patients as well.

This is important for the evaluation of the patient at the start of therapy. Patients with presumably high mortality risk should be treated immediately with a fast, comprehensive therapy (e.g. intravenous therapy for sepsis) in a suitably equipped unit (intensive care).

Early detection of patients with a high vital risk (thus also at high risk of the occurrence of organ dysfunction and other complications) is just as important for the treatment planning for patients as an early specific diagnosis (PCT as a so-called "navigation marker").

The prognostic significance of mortality-dependent measurement values (e.g. PCT, MR-pro-Adrenomedullin [MR-proADM]) should always be used to improve therapy (assignment of treatment urgency, intensified treatment, detection of high-risk patients), but not for the prediction of a final event in order to terminate therapy in the sense of a hospice situation, since even good prognostic markers are not infallible. An early, specific treatment may thus yield a favorable prognosis even for very high PCT values in a patient. The determination of progression increases the diagnostic reliability of a prognostic evaluation of PCT. Along with other clinical data, it can help to evaluate the success of therapy and to give some indication of possible changes to or retention of a therapeutic procedure.

The prognostic significance of a marker (such as PCT) has a direct influence on therapy planning: For a high vital risk, a high-quality, specific, organ-protective treatment should be started immediately, but for a lower vital risk, treatment in a normal ward under regular conditions may be warranted.

If the prognostic estimation changes over the course of treatment, this indicates the success or failure of the treatment. This may give some indication of possible changes of the treatment concept (change or discontinuing antibiotic treatment), or the need for additional diagnostic measures, e.g. a search for the focus of infection or modified therapy planning, e.g., change or discontinuing of antibiotics.

A study by Jensen et al. found a high PCT level (e.g. PCT >1 ng/ml) or an increase in PCT to be an independent predictor of the 90-day mortality in 472 critically ill patients examined (157). CRP and leukocyte counts had no prognostic significance. In an intervention study, the effectiveness of a PCT-controlled clinical intervention is currently being tested (371).

The evaluation of the necessity of antibiotic therapy is also ultimately based on an evaluation of the mortality and risk profile of the patient. For patients with a high risk profile, immediate and intensified treatment is recommended, while at a lower risk of death, a conservative, less aggressive treatment can be administered initially, or there remains time for further diagnostic clarification in the context of routine clinical diagnosis.

PCT levels can basically be interpreted as follows:

▶ Absolute values

If the PCT value is very low (with or without the presence of an infection), the patient is probably not at risk of organ dysfunction due to sepsis. Depending on the basic illness and the preceeding time-course of the disease of the patient, the mortality rate is generally low, and the acute therapeutic treatment urgency with respect to focal surgery or antibiotic treatment is relatively low.

For higher PCT levels, the picture is different. The mortality risk and thus the impetus for treatment and action are high, and an inflammatory focus requiring therapy must be assumed (usually an infection) – unless the opposite has been proved. If therapy is unsuccessful, an increased mortality risk must be assumed for the patient.

PCT influences diagnostic and therapeutic decisions:

- Low PCT values indicate a low risk of death for the patient due to severe sepsis.
- High PCT levels generally indicate a severe hazard to the patient. Therapy should be started quickly and decisively in order to treat the illness successfully.

▶ Measurement of progression (generally daily measurement)

If PCT levels fall quickly, this is generally an indication of successful treatment and a good prognosis. This is particularly true if the lower levels persist for several days and the values trend towards the normal range.

Increasing or persistently high PCT levels generally indicate continued existence of the inflammatory reaction. They are often associated with unsuccessful treatment of the patient.

The prognostic significance of PCT is generally only clear after determination of the progression:

- PCT levels which are low for several days or subside towards the normal range indicate successful treatment and a favorable prognosis (rule of thumb: a decline of more than 30% per day over at least 3 days).
- Inconsistently lowered or increasing levels, like PCT values which do not reach normal levels after several days (taking the general plasma elimination rate into consideration), can similarly indicate unsuccessful treatment or a poor prognosis.

1.7. Influence on diagnostic and therapeutic decisions during the clinical visit

Knowledge of PCT levels can have consequences for treatment, since at high levels the diagnosis of sepsis is increasingly probable, and thus fast therapy is urgent. The pre-test probability of a diagnosis of sepsis thus changes after execution of the test (☞ Figures 1.6 and 9.4). This may have therapeutic consequences, with further consequences for the prognosis and survival rate, for example an indication of immediate antibiotic therapy or fast elimination of the focus (surgery).

On the other hand, for lower PCT levels, antibiotic treatment may be avoided or discontinued under some circumstances.

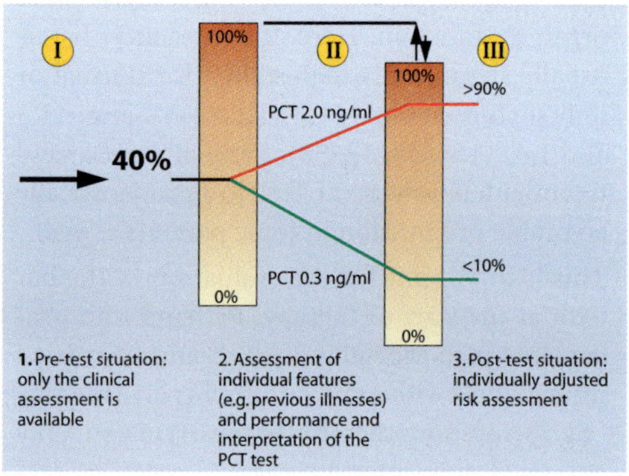

Figure 1.6: Schematic representation of the change in probability of a diagnosis with a given (estimated) pretest probability due to PCT level measurement, at different PCT levels. **1.** Clinically estimated pre-test probability of a diagnosis of sepsis or severe infection. **2.** Performance of the PCT test and integration of individual reference ranges for PCT into the interpretation (e.g. status after operation, severe liver disease). **3.** Depending on the individual circumstances and test results, the estimated probability of a diagnosis changes after administration of the test (☞ Figure 9.4).

PCT levels can be used to determine the course of activity of systemic inflammatory reactions. This information is important during the clinical visit. It gives the treating physician an indication of whether treatment is successful, whether possible complications may arise, or whether a diagnostic or therapeutic intervention should be considered. Different data is included in the evaluation of the inflammatory situation of the patient. This includes, on the one hand, less specific but sensitive values such as body temperature, leukocyte and thrombocyte counts, coagulation and other values whose plasma concentrations depend on inflammatory activity (e.g. ATIII, D-dimers, albumin). Then there are clinical data and the results of technical examination procedures (e.g. X-rays). This information should now be supplemented with measured values which react relatively specifically to bacterial infection and which reflect the severity of the inflammatory reaction (e.g. procalcitonin), in order to detect any risk to the patient quickly and to be able to act adequately (☞ Figure 1.6). Since the individual measurement values have a different diagnostic profile, a differentiated picture of the inflammatory status and risk to the patient can now be prepared, and treatment planning can be carried out ideally.

Consequences of this information, for example, include a new search for the focus of infection, changes to therapy, or indications of the effectiveness or necessity of an antibiotic treatment (☞ Sections 1.9., 6. and following). Clinical therapeutic decisions, however, should always be based on a combination of different data and observations. The single, unreflected use of PCT data for diagnostic or therapeutic purposes without precise knowledge of the patient is not recommended.

1.8. Indication and monitoring of antibiotic therapy

Different studies have shown that PCT can give indications of the necessity and duration of antibiotic therapy (22-25, 356). If one follows a few rules in the interpretation of PCT levels, the start, change, or termination of antibiotic therapy can be better adapted to the individual needs of the patient using PCT than is possible with a purely clinical estimate. This is always an evaluation of probability and risk; the individual factors of the patient and the disease must also figure in the evaluation. The estimated probability of a sepsis diagnosis and hence the need for antibiotics known to the physician after performance of the test (the post-test probability) thus rises or falls according to the PCT measurement in comparison with the pre-test probability (☞ Figure 1.6). An unnecessary, abundantly long, or ineffective treatment with antibiotics can thus be avoided.

The PCT measurement, for example, gives the physician confidence that the patient is not immediately in danger of severe sepsis at the time of PCT level measurement (in the case of low PCT levels). The changing PCT levels, in addition to the clinical data, also give an indication of whether the treatment has improved the systemic inflammatory reaction or not – with corresponding consequences for the continuation of or changes to antibiotic treatment. The measurement values determined in circulating blood, however, cannot detect whether a local wound is sufficiently well cleaned or whether the patient is still at risk from that wound. PCT can also not detect whether the patient's immune system is capable of handling the remaining infection or potential new infections without antibiotics. This must also be taken into consideration during the clinical visit in the context of infection and antibiotic monitoring. Non-specific increases in PCT, e.g. in the case of severe liver or renal insufficiency, should be included in the evaluation of levels. Numerous studies have shown that the integration of PCT into the monitoring and control of antibiotic therapy is possible and practical (☞ Chapters 6. and following).

The first studies of the control of antibiotic therapy using PCT were performed on patients with airway infections in which a significant reduction in antibiotic use was made possible with no increase in complications (22, 24). Newer studies have shown that, even in intensive care units and in patients with sepsis, severe sepsis, or pneumonia (ambulant pneumonia), a PCT-controlled individual and patient-adapted antibiotic treatment is possible. This has generally resulted in a shorter duration of treatment (23, 25, 356). More information on this topic can be found in Chapters 6. and following.

1.9. Stability and kinetics of PCT

PCT has a number of properties which support its use in the context of clinical routine. For example, PCT in blood samples is a relatively stable protein. It can be sampled for measurement together with other routinely performed blood samples, and transported to the laboratory in the usual manner, without suffering any significant decomposition (26). In the body, the clinically measurable "half-life" of the circulating inactive protein is about 24 to 35 hours (27, 28). Daily measurements in the context of the clinical visit are therefore sufficient to show changes in the plasma level for progression control or immunity monitoring. The induction period, at 4 to 12 hours, is longer than for the cytokines, but it is significantly shorter than that of CRP. Clinical conditions are generally sufficient for this period. In nearly all studies, the sensitivity and specificity values for diagnosis of sepsis are thus related to the initial or admission value in the first blood sample after the first contact with a physician or the hospital – even in the examination of children, newborns, and infants. Therefore, the notion that the induction of PCT is too slow for a rapid sepsis diagnosis – other than in a few exceptional cases – has little significance in clinical practice.

PCT in a blood sample taken under normal conditions for the handling of blood samples is a stable serum or plasma protein.
In the body, the clinical rate of decrease of elevated PCT levels (the "clinical half-life" of the calcitonin/catacalcin complex) is about 24 to 35 hours.

1.10. An overview of biochemical properties

From a biochemical standpoint, PCT is a soluble protein. It was first described as a sepsis-associated protein in 1993. It is the precursor protein for the hormone calcitonin (29). It consists of 114 to 116 amino acids (☞ Figure 1.1). In the core area of the PCT molecule is the calcitonin amino acid sequence. More detailed information about the biochemistry and pathophysiology of PCT can be found in Chapters 3. and following. The commercial PCT measurement procedures approved for clinical use detect the calcitonin/catacalcin fragment of the protein ("PCT"). The overall protein also acts as a chemokine. PCT modulates the induction of iNOS and increases mortality in animal experimental models. It inhibits the effects of CGRP at the receptor. PCT and calcitonin originate in the same gene, but their induction is regulated differently. In sepsis, different cell types and tissues produce PCT (adherent monocytary cells, liver tissue, adipocytes, if the tissue has undergone inflammatory changes), while the fragment "calcitonin" is secreted as a hormonally active peptide only by specific cells (C-cells in the thyroid and neuroendocrine cells in the lungs) (☞ Chapters 3. and following).

PCT represents a separate class of immunologically active proteins. PCT is an immune modulator which is particularly effective in clinically relevant bacterial infections. The protein can act as a chemokine and modulate different immunological functions.
PCT's structure and effect differ essentially from the cytokines, acute-phase proteins, endothelial markers, and other known immune modulators and sepsis markers.

2. Primary indications

2.1. Diagnosis, progression evaluation, and therapy of bacterial infections and sepsis

Every examination order should be based on a specific question. This applies to the request of laboratory chemical measurements as well. Such a question can either be very precise (e.g. confirmation or exclusion of a diagnosis of sepsis) or general (e.g. the use of the measured value as a screening test for monitoring of infection and sepsis in patients).

The questions associated with PCT level measurement can be very different. In the emergency room or at the physician's office, the questions about sepsis diagnosis, differential diagnostic questions, or the necessity of antibiotic treatment are in the foreground, while in the intensive care unit, the questions frequently address the evaluation of progression of systemic inflammatory reactions or the success of sepsis treatment. The monitoring or control of antibiotic therapy is also increasingly important as an indication of PCT level measurement on the ICU as well.

The most important indications for PCT level measurement can be summarized as follows:

- Diagnosis of sepsis, severe sepsis, and septic shock
- Differential diagnosis of clinically relevant bacterial infections and sepsis
- Evaluation of the severity of a bacterial infection and systemic inflammatory reactions
- Monitoring of the course of treatment of patients with sepsis
- Evaluation of progression and control of antibiotic treatment

In the following sections, general information and background will first be presented for these indications (☞ Chapter 2.), then in a specialized part (☞ Chapters 3. and following) scientific background and studies will be presented and particular indications listed.

2.1.1. Diagnosis of sepsis, severe sepsis, and septic shock

The diagnosis of sepsis, severe sepsis or septic shock can be made with greater diagnostic reliability with the use of PCT than with other laboratory chemical markers currently in use or with the exclusive use of clinical data (☞ Figures 1.6, 2.1 and 2.2).

If there is a suspicion of sepsis, the immediate PCT level measurement is recommended. Whether this is done in the physician's office, in the emergency room, in the ward, or in the intensive care unit of a hospital is unimportant. However, the diagnosis should be made quickly and decisively, and appropriate therapy should start immediately (thus ideally already in the ambulant phase, in the emergency department or in the normal ward). This is due to the fact that therapeutic measures in the initial period after the onset of "sepsis" (severe sepsis or septic shock) are most effective (30-32). If organ failure occurs, this is associated with higher mortality as severity rises (☞ Figure 1.3). PCT level measurement increases diagnostic reliability and, in many cases, leads to fast therapeutic decisions.

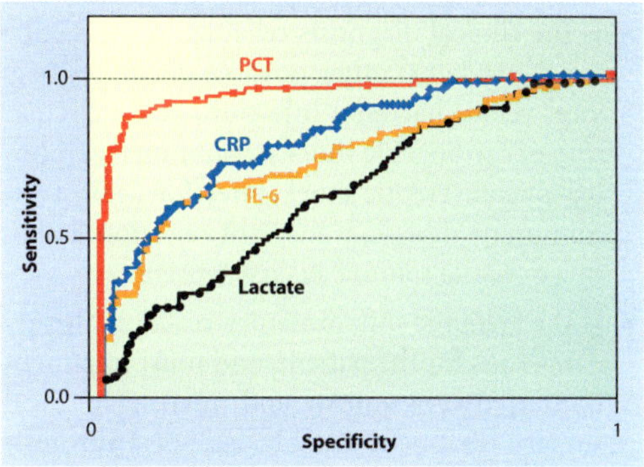

Figure 2.1: Sensitivity and specificity of PCT, CRP, IL-6, and lactate for the diagnosis of sepsis, severe sepsis, or septic shock in patients in an intensive care unit (13).

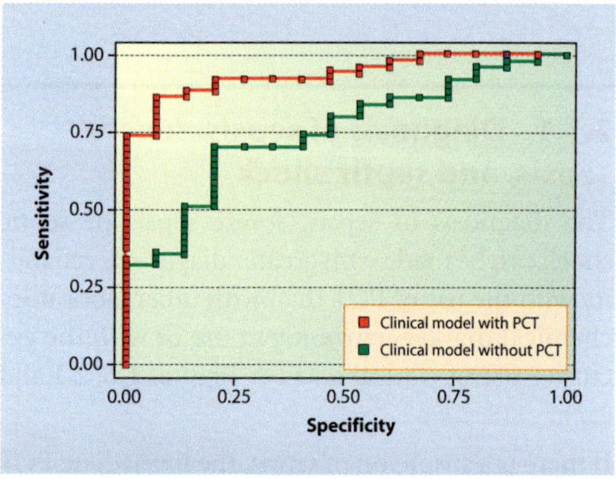

Figure 2.2: Sensitivity and specificity of a diagnosis of sepsis when using clinical data with or without consideration of procalcitonin (33).

Questions asked in the context of acute diagnosis of sepsis with PCT:

- Is there a systemic inflammatory reaction present that is already severe enough to induce PCT?
- Are the observed clinical symptoms (signs of inflammation, fever, general symptoms, any organ dysfunction, shock) associated with a bacterial infection?
- Is a quick, calculated antibiotic therapy necessary, and should there be a search for and elimination of the focus of infection?
- Is the clinical diagnosis reliable, or must it be weighed against other possible diagnoses (e.g. viral versus bacterial infection, acute circulatory or cardiogenic shock or pulmonary embolisms against septic shock, infection against autoimmune disease, transplant rejection, ischemia or tissue trauma against sepsis)?
- Is the systemic inflammatory reaction already dangerous for the patient, and must treatment be started very quickly and intensively (focal surgery, treatment with a broad-spectrum antibiotic, monitoring of organ function in the intensive care unit)?

▶ The PCT level contains a great deal of information

If PCT is very low (PCT <0.1 to under 0.25 ng/ml), the probability of the presence of a severe bacterial infection with systemic inflammation is low (high negative predictive value of very low PCT levels) (☞ Figure 1.2). The presence of an infectious bacterial disease with a high mortality risk is improbable at normal PCT levels (<0.05 ng/ml), and bacteremia is seldom expected in these patients (☞ Section 7.2.).

If the PCT level is high or very high, that information is associated with a high predictive value for the diagnosis of sepsis, severe sepsis, or septic shock (☞ Figure 1.4). High PCT levels indicate a high degree of severity of the systemic inflammatory reaction (frequent diagnosis: "severe sepsis" or "septic shock"). These are illnesses with high and increasing mortality risk. The immediate administration of an antibiotic, immediate optimization of the circulatory situation, and the rapid commencement of specific therapeutic procedures are just as essential as the rapid identification and therapy of the presumed focus of the infection (blood cultures and bacterial isolates, search for the focus of infection). Quality assurance measures should instruct and control the timely performance of intravenous therapy in every hospital (e.g. US Sepsis bundles from SCCM, sepsis benchmark (www.sepsis-benchmark.com), and mortality should be monitored (☞ e.g. www.qmits-projekt.de).

High PCT levels are always cause for alarm. Since the probability of a severe bacterial infection is high and the risk of mortality is also elevated, important and usually bacterial illnesses – depending on the clinical symptoms – must be excluded, for example bacterial pneumonia, catheter infection, pyelonephritis or urosepsis, bacterial meningitis, endocarditis, peritonitis, but also intestinal ischemia and severe pancreatitis.

For lower PCT levels, these diagnoses are also possible, but less probable – if PCT levels are low –, and generally also associated with a lower severity (e.g. for PCT levels of less than 0.1 to less than 0.25 ng/ml). PCT level measurement thus changes the diagnostic probabilities (☞ Figure 1.6). Only in very few cases is the onset of illness so acute that the time to measurable induction (generally at least 3 to 6 hours) is too short. In patients with acute symptoms and low PCT values, therefore, a follow-up measurement is recommended after 6 to 12 hours.

2.1.2. Differential diagnosis of severe bacterial infection and sepsis

Differential diagnostic decisions are also supported by PCT level measurement. In general, PCT levels are low in viral infections, allergic or autoimmune disease low, as they are in many other idiopathic inflammatory and other non-bacterial illnesses (diabetes mellitus, coronary heart disease).

Classical clinical markers of inflammation (e.g. fever or leukocyte counts) may be very sensitive and easy to measure, but they generally give few specific indications of the presence of infections. They frequently often react more feebly under immune suppression (☞ Figure 2.3). For different illnesses, extensive data has been published on the induction behavior of PCT. A selection of important diseases in which PCT level measurement plays a role can be found in Section 5.1., Table 5.1 and in Chapters 7. and following.

For differential diagnosis using PCT, experience and data is available for the following illnesses (☞ also Chapter 7. and following):

- Differentiation between viral infections and bacterial infections of various kinds (respiratory infections, pneumonia, gastroenteritis, meningitis, meningococcal infection)
- Pyelonephritis and urosepsis (in comparison with urinary tract infections)
- Pancreatitis (evaluation of severity and prognosis)
- Bacteremia
- Bacterial endocarditis
- Tropical diseases such as malaria and meloidosis and other illnesses

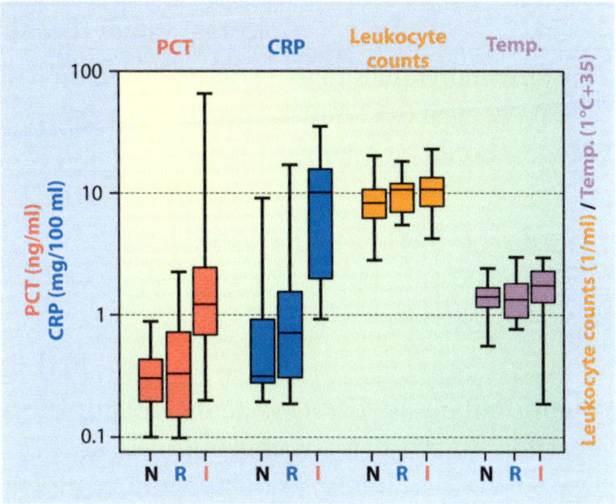

Figure 2.3: PCT, CRP, leukocyte counts (WBC), and body temperature in patients with kidney transplants with normal progression, rejection of the transplant, and infections. N = "normal progression", R = "rejection", I = "infection" (37).

▶ General guidelines for the interpretation of PCT

For the general interpretation of elevated PCT levels and their categorization in different ranges and risk categories – independent of the individual patient –, some general guidelines have been formulated (☞ Chapter 1., Table 2.1). Figure 2.4 shows some possible algorithms for clinical procedures in case of elevated PCT levels. The interpretation of values and possible clinical consequences, however, must take place in the clinical context under consideration of the individual condition of the patient. Recommendations given without knowledge of the patient (e.g. by the laboratory) must be assessed with care, since PCT, as an indirect marker of infection, can never have 100% diagnostic reliability. PCT results should therefore always be interpreted and considered in combination with all other available clinical data. An important contribution of PCT level measurement is that PCT, despite the possibility of false-negative results or non-specific induction, still detects potentially life-threatening infections with comparatively high diagnostic reliability.

The probability of a correct diagnosis of sepsis in comparison with other illnesses (e.g. cardiogenic shock, viral illnesses, autoimmune processes, pulmonary embolism) can be increased by PCT measurement in comparison with the evaluation of purely clinical or conventional data (☞ Figures 2.2 and 1.6) (33).

Normal values (healthy individuals): <0.05 ng/ml	
Healthy individuals (age ≥4 days of life); for neonates aged 0-72 hours, special reference ranges should be used (☞ Chapter 9., Figure 9.1)	Normal range for PCT (95% CI). No systemic inflammatory reaction.
PCT <0.5 ng/ml	
Measurable but low PCT response	Low or no significant systemic inflammatory reaction. Local inflammation and local infection are possible.
PCT 0.5-2.0 ng/ml	
Significant but moderate systemic inflammatory reaction. Infection is possible but there are various conditions also known to induce PCT (severe trauma, major surgery, cardiogenic shock) (☞ Chapter 8.)	Sepsis should be assumed and sepsis-specific treatment should be initiated, as long as there is no exclusion of diagnosis of sepsis or infection. If infection found: positive diagnosis of sepsis. Further PCT measurements recommended (6-24 hours)
PCT ≥2-10 ng/ml	
Severe systemic inflammatory reaction, most likely due to infection (sepsis) provided no other causes known (☞ Chapter 8.).	Diagnosis of sepsis, severe sepsis or septic shock most likely. High risk of the development of organ dysfunction. If persistently high levels (>4 days): reconsider treatment of sepsis. Possibly unfavorable prognosis. Daily measurement of PCT level recommended.
PCT ≥10 ng/ml	
Marked systemic inflammatory reaction, almost exclusively as a result of severe bacterial sepsis or septic shock	Frequently associated with organ dysfunction. High risk of fatal outcome. Daily measurement of PCT level to monitor success of treatment.

Table 2.1: General guidelines for the interpretation of PCT. PCT levels must always be interpreted in the clinical context. An isolated interpretation of PCT without knowledge of the patient should be avoided. The possibility of false-positive or false-negative reactions must be taken into consideration.

In the case of clinical suspicion of infection or sepsis despite normal PCT levels, measurements of progression should first be taken before terminating antibiotic treatment. When in doubt, we first commence anti-infective treatment until a conclusive diagnosis is available. However, if the clinical data and other standard parameters indicate no risk to the patient, antibiotic treatment can be terminated prematurely if PCT levels are normal. The fact that such a procedure is practical can also be shown for endemic meningitis (34).

▶ Special notes for a diagnosis of pneumonia

There are some special considerations for the diagnosis of pneumonia. Pneumonia is a clinical diagnosis based on the three pillars of clinical symptoms (e.g. productive cough), morphological correlation of tissue infiltration (e.g. infiltrates in the X-ray image), and different signs of inflammation (e.g. fever or leukocytosis, or even elevated PCT) and the suspicion or demonstration of an infection (if possible, with microbiological findings). An elevated PCT level is not absolutely essential for the diagnosis of pneumonia (not even for bacterial pneumonia). With elevated PCT levels, however, the diagnostic reliability for the presence of pneumonia increases if other pneumonia criteria are positive (e.g. "Clinical Pulmonary Infection Score", CPIS) (383). With elevated PCT levels, therefore, there must also be some reason to consider pneumonia as a possible focus of infection. Elevated PCT levels especially occur in severe pneumonia or pneumonia with a high mortality risk and with a bacterial cause, while viral or other causes (mycoplasma) and bacterial pneumonia with less severity or lower mortality risk need not be associated with elevated PCT levels. An elevated

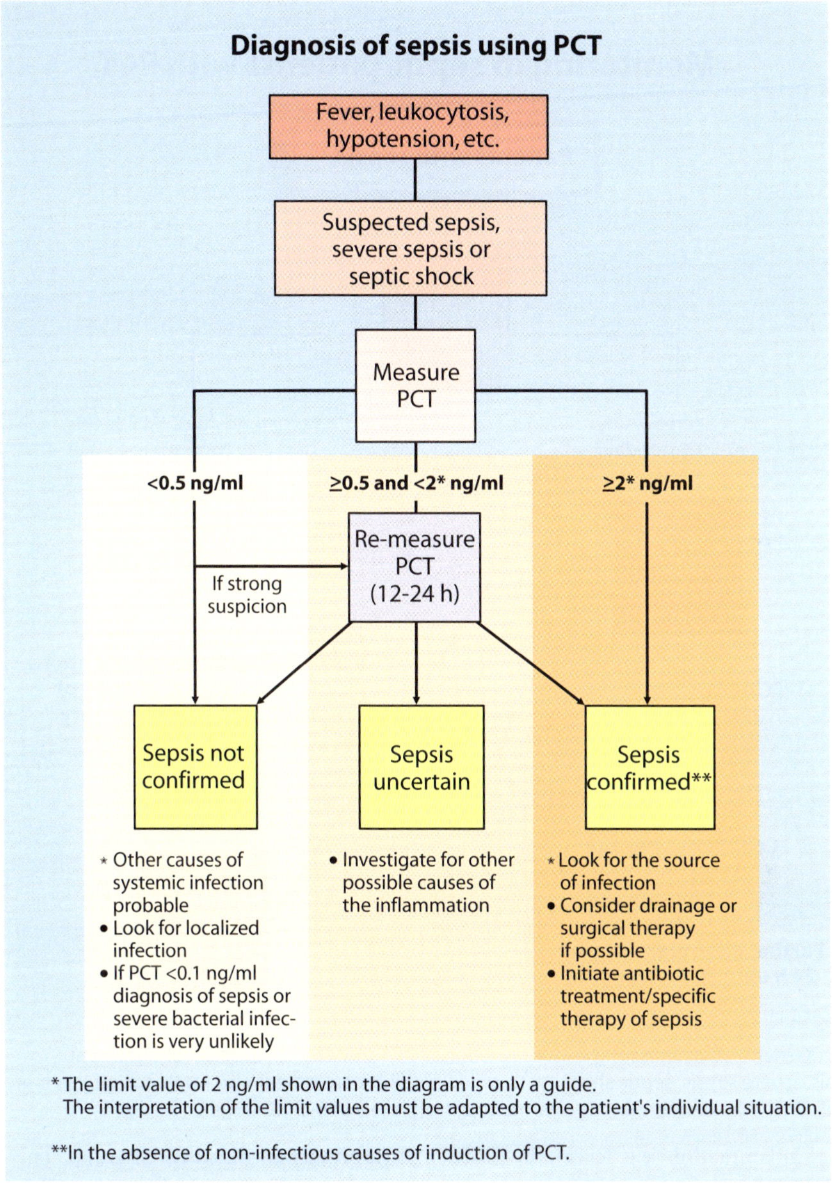

Figure 2.4: General guidelines for the interpretation of elevated PCT values when there is a suspicion of sepsis. PCT levels must always be interpreted in the clinical context.

PCT level in pneumonia can also be used to evaluate the success of treatment or evaluation of risk of infection (e.g. as an indication of a severe progression with sepsis, severe sepsis, or septic shock and hence for the duration and effectiveness of antibiotic therapy) (☞ Section 5.2. and 6.2.) (20, 35, 36).

Finally, note that one should not forget to take isolates (e.g. blood samples, sputum) before initiating antibiotic therapy to allow for microbiological examination and/or determination of possible bacterial causes. However, this should not delay the commencement of treatment. More frequently than in other patients, blood cultures are positive with elevated PCT levels. Patients with bacteremia, on average, have higher PCT levels than patients without bacteremia (☞ Section 7.2.) Conversely, for very low PCT levels, even with clinically posi-

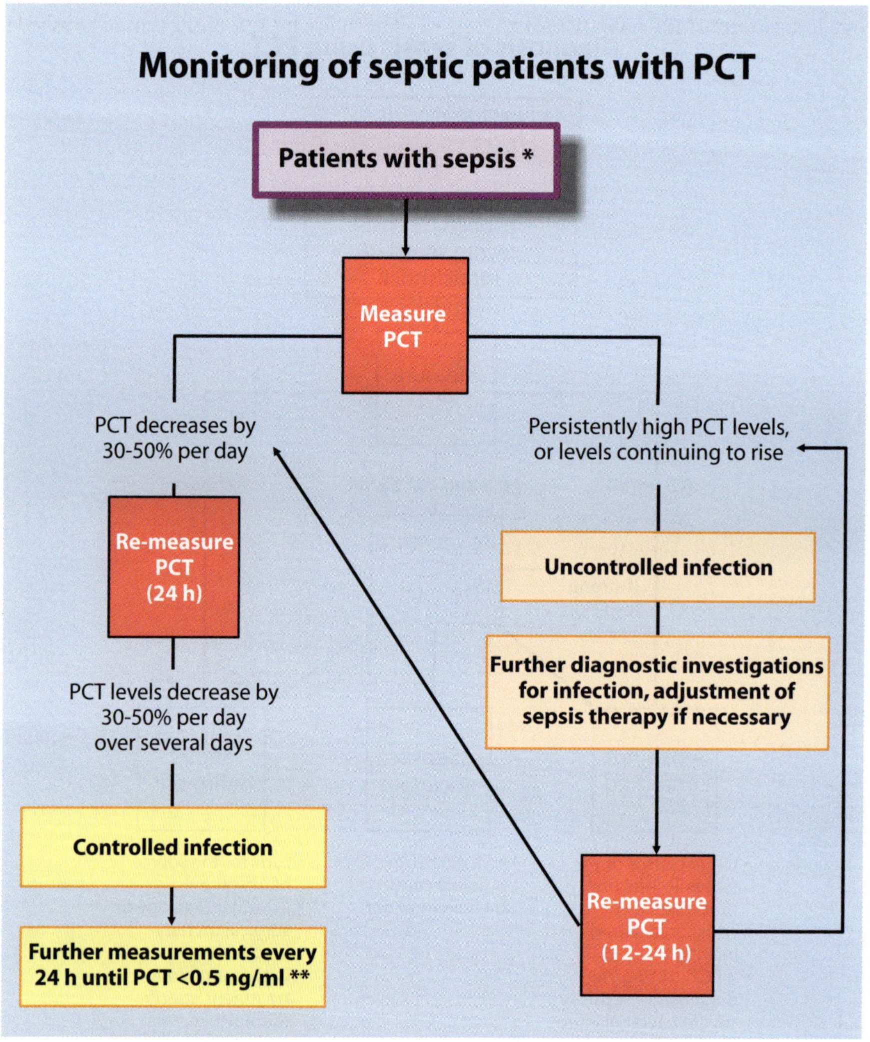

Figure 2.5: General guidelines for the interpretation of PCT trends after the start of treatment.
* here sepsis, severe sepsis, septic shock; ** To guide antibiotic treatment also lower cut-off levels are used. For more details on guidance of antibiotic treatment, cut-off levels and algorithms ☞ Section 6.

tive signs of inflammation (e.g. fever), the probability of the presence of positive blood cultures is low. Especially for elevated PCT levels, we should therefore consider a blood culture or performance of a microbial PCR.

2.1.3. Evaluation of the severity of sepsis and the systemic inflammatory reaction

In addition to strengthening the diagnosis of a severe bacterial infection or sepsis, the evaluation of the current severity of the systemic inflammatory response of the observed clinical picture is of great importance in the acute situation. This information has a significant influence on the diagnostic and therapeutic procedure: a highly severe systemic inflammatory activation implies a high risk of the occurrence of organ dysfunction. It requires fast, decisive action, since mortality is directly related to the degree of organ dysfunction (☞ Figure 1.3). Only a fast, successful therapy can generally prevent the progression of organ dysfunction (focal surgery, antibiotic therapy, optimization of hemodyamics and tissue perfusion, and, if necessary, a sepsis-specific therapy).

PCT gives indications of the severity of the systemic inflammatory response:

- High PCT levels are often found in conjunction with severe sepsis or septic shock; the risk of organ dysfunction is high.
- Low PCT levels indicate a lower activation of the systemic inflammatory response. There is usually no bacterial infection causing the inflammation, or there is only a local bacterial infection with mild systemic inflammatory components. The vital threat of infection is low.
- In any case, the possibility of false-positive and false-negative results must be taken into consideration when interpreting PCT levels.

If PCT is elevated in an individual case and no bacterial infection can be found, one should preferably pursue antibiotic treatment, since these patients are often severely ill and their immune defenses weakened. The risk of bacterial translocation and other secondary infections is generally high.

The following explanations may serve as a general guideline for the evaluation of elevated PCT levels (☞ Figure 2.5; see also the details of the FDA approval in the United States in Section 1.4.):

PCT levels from 0.5 ng/ml to over 2 ng/ml indicate, with increasing probability, the presence of a severe bacterial infection or sepsis. In patients with severe kidney or liver dysfunction or after a trauma (the first few days after an operation or accidental trauma), values of 0.5 ng/ml to 2 ng/ml can be seen as normal, however. In this case, evaluation of the progression is important. In most algorithms guiding antibiotic therapy, for a high level of security, a threshold ≥0.25 ng/ml PCT is recommended to initiate or to continue antibiotic therapy.

PCT levels of more than 2 ng/ml or over 10 ng/ml should be considered high to very high. The probability of diagnosis of sepsis, severe sepsis, or septic shock is high (generally higher than 90% to 98%). Such values are generally signs of a severe systemic inflammatory response with the threat of, or already progressing, organ dysfunction (☞ Figure 2.4).

The following questions should be asked in conjunction with the interpretation of PCT and the presumed severity of the illness:

- Are therapeutic efforts appropriate for the high risk to the patient (e.g. intensive care, broad spectrum antibiotic therapy, extensive search for the focus of infection, protective measures for the organs)?
- Can the observed PCT levels be explained by the current diagnosis being treated?
- How elevated are the PCT values, and thus how high is the risk of additional complications (e.g. organ dysfunction)?
- Is the cause of the PCT elevation known (e.g. bacterial infection)?
- Is the treatment effective (start checking progression!)?
- Are there other reasons for the observed PCT elevation (e.g. non-bacterial causes such as organ necrosis, rhabdomyolysis, pancreatitis, fungal infections, or heat shock)?

2.1.4. Progression and prognostic significance

The most frequent application of PCT measurements in the intensive care unit is to evaluate the progression of sepsis and severe bacterial infections. This has an influence on the possible additional diagnostic and therapeutic measures. PCT level measurement can provide indications for the prognosis of the illness and the individual risk to the patient. Indications of the necessity or effectiveness of an antibiotic treatment are also obtained.

From the progression of PCT levels, we can draw conclusions about the success of therapy or the prognosis of the illness. Increases in PCT must be seen as an indication of a possible infection, while decreasing or normal PCT values are often an indication of a successful therapy or the end of a severe infection (157, 372). In new onsets of fever, PCT can provide indications of sepsis or bacterial infection as a possible cause (372).

PCT can be used over the course of the illness to determine the progression or decrease of the systemic inflammatory response. This information is often indirectly related to the success of the therapy. An evaluation of the progression is thus a focus of the

PCT measurement. In hospitals working with PCT, the majority of PCT measurements made are used for quantitative determinations of progression. PCT is a part of their daily routine diagnostics. Different questions may represent an indication for daily PCT measurement in certain patients. These include questions about the control and evaluation of treatment, the observation or monitoring of patients, and prognostic questions and questions about the planning of additional diagnostic or therapeutic intervention.

PCT level measurement trends can thus describe the activity of the inflammatory response over the course of the illness, evaluate the effectiveness of a current treatment (antibiotic therapy, focal elimination), detect new complications ("immune monitoring"), offer support for decisions about the necessity for further interventions (e.g. relaparotomy, a change in antibiotic, termination or reinforcement of therapy), or enable a careful prognostic evaluation.

A fast decline in PCT levels within the first few days of the start of treatment is often an indication of a good prognosis, while steady or increasing PCT levels often result in a mortality outcome of the disease (12, 20, 36, 38-40).

Trend measurements support clinical decisions in the following questions:

- When starting therapy:
  - Is the current therapy effective?
  - Must the therapy be corrected?
  - Is the diagnosis correct, or should it be reconsidered?
- Over the course of the illness:
  - Is the systemic inflammatory process under control?
  - Should a new search for the focus of infection or focal surgery be performed?
  - Is persistent inflammation delaying the healing process (change of infectious agent, resistant infectious agents, fungal infections, or hospital diseases)?
  - Are antibiotics used effectively or can antibiotic treatment be discontinued?

Daily monitoring of PCT in risk patients provides indications of the progression of the systemic inflammatory response (e.g. when antibiotics are stopped). This contributes to an increase in diagnostic reliability, since newly occurring severe sepsis can be detected with a higher probability than with purely clinical observation.

The question often arises as to which patients in an intensive care unit should be monitored with daily PCT measurements.

In addition to patients for whom PCT levels help evaluate the initial success of therapy (e.g. the effectiveness of an antibiotic treatment, or focal surgery for sepsis), this is especially directed to patients in whom septic complications might arise over the course of the therapy ("infection monitoring", e.g. after termination of antibiotic therapy) – although PCT cannot detect every new infection (e.g. pneumonia, catheter infection, infection of external ventricle drainages). Here, infection monitoring must include additional clinical signs, indications of a local infection, and other specific determinations.

The following intensive care patients should receive immune monitoring with PCT:

- All patients with antibiotic therapy to check the effectiveness of treatment.
- Patients in whom therapy pauses or termination of antibiotic therapy is ordered (daily measurement).
- Patients at increased risk for sepsis or severe infections (e.g. due to general accompanying illnesses, immobilization, compromised immune function, injuries, operations) (here, daily measurement is recommended).
- Patients for whom treatment or monitoring of a focus of infection is required (control of therapeutic success, e.g. in soft tissue injuries, peritonitis, pneumonia).
- Patients receiving long-term ventilation (with the risk of pneumonia and other hospital-associated infections).
- Patients with venous or arterial catheters of any kind (risk of catheter-associated infections).
- Patients subject to immune suppression (oncology, transplantation, chemotherapy, neutropenia).

- Postoperative or post-traumatic patients (general surgery, traumatology, risk of insufficient anastomosis, wound or soft tissue infections), if there is any increased risk of infection or sepsis suspected.
- Patients at increased risk of superinfections (burns, viral infections).
- Patients with nonspecific diagnostic pictures or lacking diagnoses.

Moreover, PCT also has good prognostic characteristics. The progression of PCT levels allows for indications of the prognosis of the illness. Note that the absolute value of the initial PCT level has only limited prognostic significance. With proper treatment, even highly elevated PCT levels need not represent an extraordinarily high mortality risk if the underlying disease is quickly cured. This is often the case, for example, with acute pyelonephritis or early urosepsis, where extremely high PCT levels are observed initially, which quickly decrease after effective antibiotic therapy.

Much more important than the absolute level of PCT is the trend of the levels after the start of treatment. If concentrations do not fall rapidly, or if they fail to reach the expected base level within the anticipated period of treatment (taking the clinical half-life and individual situation of the patient into consideration), this is generally a bad prognostic sign. In clinical practice, the prognostic evaluation of PCT levels is not often used to address the question of possible termination of therapy, but rather to examine the ongoing therapeutic procedure in accordance with the presumed prognosis and to introduce or eliminate further diagnostic or therapeutic steps as necessary.

2.1.5. Indication and control of antibiotic treatment

The information provided by PCT gives indications of the possible necessity of antibiotic treatment (particularly for outpatients or in the emergency room, in the case of suspected bacterial airway infections, or for suspected cases of sepsis).

After starting antibiotic treatment, the progression of the systemic inflammatory response can be described by PCT. This is often an indication of the effectiveness of treatment. Further, duration of antibiotic therapy can be better adapted to the individual needs of the patient if a PCT-based algorithm is used. It was shown in various studies that by applying such algorithm the antibiotic therapy could be reduced by more than 2 days on the average (☞ Chapter 6., Table 6.2).This data can also be used in the intensive care unit – in combination with other, usually clinical, information – to improve the adaptation of the effectiveness and possible duration of treatment to the individual patient (23, 25).

Since questions about the indication of antibiotic therapy or control of antimicrobial treatment are generally very specific, please refer to the appropriate sections (☞ Section 2.2.1., PCT in the intensive care unit; Chapters 6. and following, airway infections; Section 7.1., PCT in pneumonia).

Summary

An important indication for PCT level measurement is the progression of an infection or sepsis to severe sepsis or septic shock. This results in different applications, including differential diagnosis in comparison with non-bacterial inflammatory illnesses. Different independent examinations and meta-analyses have confirmed these indications (a high degree of evidence-based medicine).

Over the course of the illness, PCT can provide indications of the progression of the inflammatory activation of the disease, and thus contribute indirectly to the prognosis or success of treatment.

A control of the application of antibiotic therapy and monitoring of its therapeutic success is also possible by means of PCT. Therapeutic decisions, however, should include clinical data in the evaluation. The individual clinical situation must be taken into consideration. Various studies have shown that PCT permits antibiotic treatment adapted individually to the patient and the risk of illness. This procedure, due to extensive general use of antibiotics and the high rate of resistant germs, is obviously preferable to a rigid treatment schema.

2.2. PCT level measurement in specific clinical areas

2.2.1. PCT in the intensive care unit

Daily work with PCT levels and their interpretation are of great importance for physician rounds in the intensive care unit. In combination with other measured values, PCT can provide information about the functional organ system, the "systemic inflammatory response". If the results of different inflammation-activated measurement values are combined, taking their specific characteristics into consideration (e.g. PCT, leukocyte counts, body temperature, trends in coagulation parameters including thrombocyte counts and other measured values), PCT can provide the consulting physician with information about the progression and severity of the systemic inflammatory response, which is primarily the consequence of a bacterial infection. This information, like knowledge about the progression of organ dysfunction, has an influence on therapy. For example, after complex intestinal surgery with an initial suspicion of sepsis and peritonitis, falling signs of inflammation can quickly initiate a routine treatment plan, while in case of "increasing" or "highly active" signs of inflammation, a broadly effective antibiotic therapy, specific therapeutic procedures, the question of peritonitis or insufficient anastomosis and even the necessity of a repeated intervention should be discussed.

PCT levels are often used in the context of daily routine laboratory examinations in intensive care units for determination of progression and the infection/inflammation monitoring of high-risk patients.

Even in the intensive care unit, antibiotic therapy can be better adapted to the individual needs and risks of the patient with measured PCT levels than without the knowledge of infection/inflammation-related values.

The individual questions in the specific case can determine which patients should be subject to PCT level measurement.

▶ What should specifically be taken into consideration in the intensive care unit?

In the intensive care unit, the question of a non-bacterial PCT induction is more frequent. Even for falling PCT levels after focal surgery, not all patients reach the normal range of less than 0.05 ng/ml in healthy subjects within a given time. Possible causes of the non-bacterial induction of PCT should therefore be known (☞ Sections 8.1. through 8.5.). Generalized activation of the immune system or organic perfusion ("microcirculation abnormalities") can also sometimes cause a (usually moderate) increase in PCT without any evidence of a specific bacteria focus, if weakened intestinal barrier functions lead to "bacterial translocation".

Patients with septic shock, for example, often exhibit bacteremia (3). However, in these cases the search for a focus should not be omitted (possible sources of infection: catheter infection, pneumonia, urinary tract infection, endocarditis, bacteremia, and others). For immune-suppressed patients and patients undergoing chemotherapy, special conditions apply for the interpretation of PCT.

▶ In which intensive care patients should PCT be measured?

As a rule, even in the intensive care unit, PCT should only be measured in selected patients and to answer specific questions. The indications listed above apply (☞ Section 2.1., Chapters 5., 7. and following).

The following questions are often good cause for PCT level measurement in the intensive care unit:

- A control of the effectiveness of a focal surgery or antibiotic treatment:
  - PCT levels should be measured at the outset and during the course of an antibiotic treatment. The daily trend then indicates how PCT is reacting to the treatment. Under some circumstances, it is possible to skip a day of measurement if there are no therapeutic or diagnostic decisions planned for the following day (for possible consequences, see below). Thus, effectiveness and duration of antibiotic therapy can be assessed.

  - During treatment of or after surgery for an infectious/inflammatory focus, the effectiveness of the treatment should be checked using PCT (e.g. for peritonitis, after an intestinal resection, in soft tissue infections or amputations in patients with weakened microperfusion, pAVK, or diabetes).
- Performance of inflammation/infection monitoring (in combination with other signs of infection) for better detection of new sepsis or infections:
  - In patients with a general risk of possible hospital infections (e.g. during longer periods of intensive care due to neurological deficiencies, patients with acute, severe cerebral damage, pre-rehabilitation phase)
  - For the monitoring of patients at higher risk of infection due to specific illnesses (patients with extensive soft tissue injury, soft tissue injury with weakened microcirculation, polytraumatized patients, patients with weakened immune function).
  - For patients who no longer need any (specific) antibiotic therapy (see below). Prophylactic antibiotic therapy or treatment cycles with antibiotics beyond 7 days should always be avoided, even in intensive care units. Patients who are not receiving antibiotics due to this strategy should be monitored with a daily PCT level measurement. If PCT levels rise (and if there are other indications of possible infection), then a search for the focus and, if necessary, antibiotic treatment, should follow.
- Differential diagnostic questions and confirmation or exclusion of a diagnosis of sepsis:
  - These questions usually arise at the start of intensive medical treatment. There are numerous cases in which a misdiagnosis by the admitting department could be quickly corrected based on a PCT level measurement.
  - Even in the case of an unexpected increase in PCT levels, the question of a new case of sepsis must be discussed. A search for the focus and a corresponding rapid diagnosis and treatment are recommended.

▶ Monitoring of antibiotic therapy in the intensive care unit

Given sufficient experience with the interpretation of PCT, the marker can be used along with other clinical measurements in the intensive care unit as well to monitor or control antibiotic therapy (25, 356). A detailed explanation of this indication can be found in Chapter 6., especially in Sections 6.2.4. through 6.3.. This means that PCT can provide an indication of the possible effectiveness of an anti-infective therapy. If PCT levels decrease rapidly after treatment is started, it is generally unnecessary to change an antibiotic therapy (while taking the microbial findings and clinical data into consideration), since this is an indication of successful treatment or a prognostically favorable progression of the illness. If the levels fail to decrease, this is more frequently associated with an unfavorable prognosis, and the current therapy and diagnosis should be reexamined (157). If the clinical symptoms indicate healing or disappearance of an infection, low PCT values can be an additional argument for discontinuing antibiotic treatment. This is often the case as early as the 5th to 7th day of treatment. If these patients remain in intensive care for other reasons but no longer receive antibiotics, then in addition to clinical monitoring, immune monitoring using PCT should be done in order to detect possible septic complications or severe opportunistic infections quickly during the further progression.

2.2.2. PCT in the emergency room

In the emergency room, acute diagnostics are the top priority. It must be decided quickly whether a patient has sepsis or how urgent treatment is. Evaluation of the mortality risk to the patient is essential: given indications of a vital hazard to the patient (a high risk of mortality), intensified, goal-oriented treatment must be started immediately (e.g. intravenous treatment for sepsis in intensive care, rapid treatment of the focus, immediate organ-protective therapy). Possible differential diagnoses must be made. If the mortality risk is low, treatment in the context of the usual routine is generally sufficient.

Diagnostic markers such as PCT and MR-pro-ADM provide the physician with an improved evaluation of mortality risk. They also provide indications for special diagnoses (e.g. sepsis). This increases the probability of the correct treatment, and the physician is warned about possible underestimation of dangerous risks (e.g. delayed treatment of the patient due to underestimation of the severity of the disease, unjustified or incorrect treatment in the normal ward).

In addition, so-called "navigation markers", which provide specific indications of typical diseases, improve the early stages of diagnosis and therapy (e.g. D-dimers for pulmonary embolism and thrombosis, PCT for sepsis, MR-proANP, NT-proBNP or MR-proADM for acute heart failure, S100 and NSE for cerebral damage, troponin for myocardial infarct).

The PCT measurement value can provide an indication of whether sepsis is present or not, whether a bacterial inflammatory focus may exist, and whether a clinically relevant systemic inflammatory response is endangering the patient. By measuring PCT levels, therefore, the perceived risk of the presence of severe bacterial infection of sepsis in the patient changes (☞ Figure 1.6). PCT also permits the evaluation of patient risk with respect to mortality and success of treatment (prognostic characteristics of PCT).

The exclusion of possible sepsis, e.g. in case of unsure suspicion of cardiogenic shock, pulmonary embolism, dehydration, or meningitis, is often a reason for PCT level measurement in the emergency room.

Differential diagnostic decisions, evaluation of patient risk, and increased reliability of a diagnosis of sepsis are often indications for PCT level measurement in the emergency room. Additional indications and differential diagnoses are presented in Section 2.1.2. and Chapters 7. and following.

The following diseases are often causes of elevated PCT levels and sepsis in the emergency room:

- Sepsis in
  - Peritonitis (cause: perforation of a hollow organ, intestinal ischemia)
  - Pneumonia
  - Pyelonephritis, urinary tract infections
  - Bacteremia
  - Soft tissue infections and abscesses
  - Gastroenteritis
  - Meningitis
  - Aspiration
- Possible differential diagnoses which can simulate sepsis include:
  - Nonspecific neurological altered status of consciousness
  - Hemodynamic instability (cardiogenic shock, pulmonary embolism)
  - Nonspecific fever (viral infection, local bacterial infection)
  - Nonspecific abdominal symptoms (note: in acute appendicitis or cholecystitis, there may be no significant elevation of PCT levels if there is no extensive peritonitis or perforation)

The measurement of multiple highly specific markers (e.g. D-dimers, MR-proADM, NT-ProNBP/MR-proANP/ProBNP, troponin, and so on) can improve diagnostic reliability from a laboratory standpoint.

In the emergency room, it is essential to set a course rapidly. Misdiagnoses and delayed diagnoses should be avoided where possible. PCT increases the diagnostic reliability and, in comparison with other measured values, has a high sensitivity and specificity for the diagnosis of sepsis. In the emergency room, PCT helps improve the diagnosis of bacterial infections (372, 373). PCT permits improved estimation of patient risk (risk of mortality) (157, 370). Elevated or rising PCT levels are associated with an increased mortality risk (157, 370, 373).

The significance of a rapid therapy with a time window of a few hours is shown by the publication of Kumar et al. (30). Here, the mortality rate of patients with septic shock was examined retrospectively for intensive care units in the United States and Canada with respect to the start of therapy (administration of the correct antibiotic). Mortality increased an average of 7% per hour when the start of therapy was delayed. Commencement of therapy later than 24 to 48 hours after admission is generally no longer effective. Rapid therapy also preserves the resources of a hospital, since early treatment of sepsis is less costly and therefore economically more favorable than treatment of advanced forms of the disease with organ dysfunction. Treatment includes, on the one hand, antibiotic therapy and elimination of the focus and, on the other hand, the immediate stabilization of the circulation and, if necessary, the use of specific supportive therapeutic measures, such as the administration of recombinant human-activated protein C.

Given this data, the use of a diagnostic marker that significantly increases the reliability of the initial diagnosis should be essential. In various studies of the diagnosis of sepsis, severe sepsis, or septic shock, PCT had a sensitivity and specificity of over 80%, sometimes greater than 90%. These values do depend on the circumstances and the patient population examined (pre-test probability). However, practical experience and different meta-analyses show that these results are evidence-based (41-43).

Immediate therapy is essential for the course of the disease and mortality of the illness in sepsis, severe sepsis, or septic shock. Fast diagnosis is therefore very important.

In the emergency room, the use of a laboratory chemical marker with high sensitivity and specificity for the diagnosis of sepsis and detection of severe systemic inflammatory response (such as procalcitonin) should be taken for granted in the context of initial diagnosis.

▶ What are the consequences in the emergency room, if the exact diagnosis is unknown?

If PCT levels cannot be assigned to a specific diagnosis, the clinical impression remains the deciding factor. As a general guide to interpretation, patients with currently normal PCT levels are very probably not in danger of severe sepsis. If the suspicion of sepsis is clinically supported despite negative PCT values, sepsis therapy should initially be started and the search for a focus continued. PCT levels should be measured again after 2 to 6 hours, until a final diagnosis is obtained (☞ Figure 2.4).

This applies to any antibiotic treatment as well. If the clinical impression permits, a low PCT level may support a decision against antibiotic treatment, since it is an indication of a low risk of severe infection or organ dysfunction as the consequence of bacterial infection. For elevated PCT levels, even for clinically less remarkable patients, a diagnosis of sepsis or severe infection, and thus antibiotic therapy, should be considered. If there is an urgent clinical suspicion of sepsis or severe infection despite a negative PCT result, the clinical impression should always be taken into consideration, since PCT can also give false-negative results. That means that an antibiotic treatment should be started.

If the final diagnosis cannot be clarified even with the aid of a PCT level measurement, the usual diagnostic or therapeutic steps traditionally used in the clinic should determine the further course of action.

Examples of use

- A 50-year-old patient presents in the clinic with abdominal symptoms (pressure pain in the upper right abdomen). A sonogram shows a mild thickening of the wall of the gall bladder. A tentative diagnosis of cholecystitis is made. If PCT levels are elevated (e.g. PCT above 2 ng/ml), the operation should be performed immediately. Peritonitis and organ dysfunction are possible. If PCT levels are normal, on the other hand, admission of the patient to the regular OP schedule on a timely basis is possible.

- A 68-year-old patient presents with cardiac arrhythmia, borderline hypotonic blood pressure values, and an overall weakened condition (gray skin coloration, cold sweat). Within the next 24 hours, the patient requires catecholamine in the intensive care unit. The patient has a history of a heart valve defect of medium severity, with restricted pump function. A diagnosis of progredient cardiogenic shock is made. As the patient's need for catecholamine increases, PCT levels are measured retrospectively. An initial PCT value of 4 ng/ml at admission is determined. At this point, the patient's circulation was essentially still stable, she was breathing spontaneously, and was catecholamine-free. The PCT levels rise quickly to more than 10 ng/ml. Although an echocardiogram shows no indication of increasing valvular dysfunction or endocarditis, the patient is treated with antibiotics and quickly moved to a cardiac surgery unit. After another 24 hours at this unit, the patient is diagnosed with endocarditis and surgery is performed on the patient immediately. The diagnosis is surgically confirmed.

- An 18-year-old patient presents with recurring nausea and pain in the lower right abdomen. PCT levels are normal. Clinically, appendicitis is suspected. An appendectomy is performed on the same day, since the diagnosis of appendicitis must be made independently of the PCT level.
- A 25-year-old patient presents with the same symptoms. The PCT level is elevated, at 2 ng/ml. Here, too, an immediate appendectomy is performed. A perforation of the appendix with peritonitis is discovered. To monitor the course of the disease, PCT levels are measured daily in order to detect successful treatment of the illness, both clinically and chemically. Since the PCT levels continue to decrease daily – in combination with other findings, which are also unremarkable –,the antibiotic treatment can be discontinued after a few days.
- A 30-year-old patient with a 5-day history of continuing diarrhea despite administration of antibiotics is admitted to the emergency room with cold sweats. He reports coming to the hospital due to increasing weakness and asthenia. Besides nonspecific abdominal symptoms, clinical examination reveals no indication of specific symptoms, and electrolyte levels are normal. However, laboratory chemistry shows leukopenia. The PCT level, however, is 20 ng/ml. Due to suspicion of sepsis, an immediate intravenous calculated antibiotic therapy and fluid therapy is started. Over the next few hours, he quickly exhibits the beginnings of organ failure, decreasing thrombocyte counts, and coagulation deficiency. A diagnosis of severe sepsis with gastroenteritis is made, and therapy with recombinant human protein C is started immediately. The patient survives with no permanent injury.

2.2.3. PCT in outpatient cases

In the future, PCT will be used more frequently in outpatient care. Simpler, faster measurement procedures, along with the use of the test as an indicator for or against immediate antibiotic treatment – in addition to classical indications of a diagnosis of sepsis – are leading to the use of PCT as an emergency or routine parameter in outpatient practice. There are scientific studies supporting the use of PCT in the physician's office. Thus, it will be practical in the future to measure PCT more frequently in outpatient care in order to reduce the necessity for prescription of antibiotics, but also because patients with a diagnosis of "sepsis" are not recognised in outpatient care despite the "clinical view" (☞ Table 2.2).

Different studies show that the use of PCT can also significantly reduce the rate of prescription of antibiotics in outpatient care (☞ Figure 2.6) (22, 24, 44). This is important not only due to cost or possible side effects, but also because it is known that the frequency of occurrence of resistant agents depends on the frequency of use of antibiotics (45-47) (☞ Figure 6.1).

Since fast, reliable PCT level measurement is becoming simpler for outpatient care as well, the significance of these measurement values in outpatient care is growing.

▶ Patient- and risk-adapted antibiotic therapy for infection illnesses treated on an outpatient basis

In a multi-center study in Switzerland, in which 53 practicing physicians participated and 458 patients could be included, the rate of prescription of antibiotics could be reduced by 72% with no increase in days of illness (☞ Figure 2.6) (PARTI study) (44). Note that in Switzerland, in comparison with other countries, relatively few antibiotics are prescribed (☞ Figures 6.1 and 6.2) (46, 47). A significant reduction in the rate of prescription was achieved in bronchitis, laryngotracheitis, tonsillitis, and exacerbated COPD (☞ also Sections 6.1. through 6.2.4.).

▶ Evaluation of systemic inflammatory response and the severity of bacterial infections in physician's offices

Of course, PCT can also provide indications of local or systemic bacterial infections in outpatient care. For a normal or very low PCT level (<0.1 ng/ml), the diagnosis of severe sepsis is nearly excluded (high negative predictive value of PCT). However, mildly elevated PCT levels of more than 0.1 ng/ml can be observed in up to a tenth of the cases with no infection present – especially for older patients or patients with preexisting conditions (e.g. kidney disease) (48). Conversely, for simple local infections, PCT shows no reaction in many patients. PCT should therefore not be used as a screening test for bacterial local infections, but rather as a measurement indicating

Reason for treatment	Examples	Selection of antibiotic	Duration of treatment	PCT-controlled use
"Convenience" (symptom reduction, less pain, shorter duration of treatment)	Enteritis, bronchitis, laryngitis, tracheitis pharyngitis, rhinosinusitis, sometimes urinary tract infection	As little antibiosis as possible. As little broadly effective antibiotic treatment as possible.	None. Short and symptom-oriented, if necessary.	Yes, to exclude the necessity for therapy. (Exclusion of sepsis). Evidence basis: yes.
Lack of self-limitation of the illness, threat of spreading, dangerous agent.	Otitis externa, endocarditis, urinary tract infections, erysipelas, different soft tissue infections, tuberculosis	Calculated antibiotic therapy, if possible with a specific, less broadly-effective antibiotic. Attempt identification of agent. Special case: tuberculosis.	Sometimes temporary (urinary tract infection, otitis externa), sometimes over longer time (endocarditis, tuberculosis)	Not necessary. If necessary to determine the end of therapy. Evidential basis weak.
Locally destructive processes	Endocarditis, arthritis, infection of cerebrospinal fluid drainages, infection of metallic implants, pyelonephritis. Tonsillitis if A-streptococcus found, tuberculosis	If possible, isolation of agent and selection of a specific, tissue-penetrating antibiotic.	Until healed. Frequently, surgical intervention required and antibiotic therapy only accompanying. In special cases, until eradication of the agent (streptococcus, Tbc).	Not needed in all cases if diagnosis known. If necessary to determine end of treatment. However, there are no clinical data or study data available. (Not evaluated).
Suspicion of sepsis, severe sepsis, or septic shock	Pneumonia with sepsis, peritonitis, urosepsis, acute abdominal and other infection sources	Immediate start of treatment (calculated antibiotic therapy) with a broad spectrum antibiotic	Until the systemic inflammatory response has subsided and the focus has been eliminated.	Yes, to reinforce or exclude a diagnosis of sepsis and to monitor progression (monitoring of effectiveness and end of treatment) Evidential basis: high. In case of clinical suspicion: or high PCT levels: immediate start of therapy. Confirmation with PCT later. After reliable exclusion of diagnosis or end of sepsis (focal intervention) discontinue antibiotics. When in doubt, clinical data takes precedence until a final diagnosis is known.

Table 2.2: Possible reasons for the prescription of antibiotics, examples of corresponding diseases and pointers for possibly rational measurement of PCT in association with corresponding diagnostic investigations and treatment. If antibiotics are prescribed, the reason for the prescription should always be known to the physician (Record the suspected diagnosis!). This is a good tool to evaluate the need or the necessary duration of treatment and to make a decision as to whether monitoring of the treatment with PCT level measurement would be beneficial. The presumed reason for the illness also influences the selection of antibiotics used.

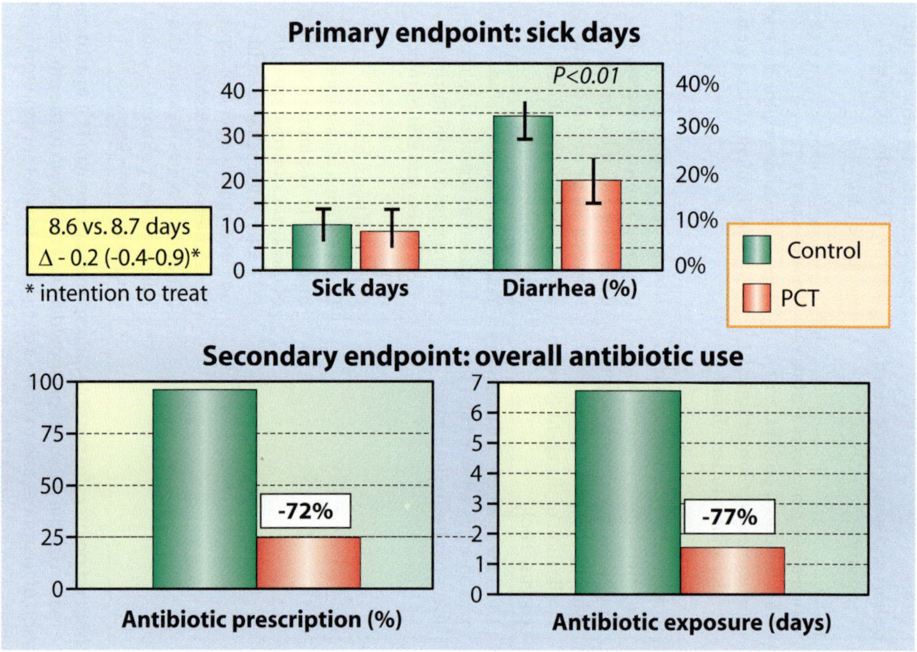

Figure 2.6: Effects of PCT-controlled antibiotic therapy in outpatient care. The rate of prescription of antibiotics, the rate of diarrheal illness, and the total duration of antibiotic exposure are reduced, while the number of days of illness does not increase. Number of patients, n = 458. After (44).

systemic inflammatory response as the consequence of an infection (e.g. sepsis) or a severe bacterial infection.

For normal PCT values, local infections can still be present as well. If these have locally destructive consequences or affect at-risk organs (e.g. infected ventricle drainage, threat of miscarriage, endoprostheses), therapy must be started quickly, even if there is no sepsis. It is thus important for the treating physician to be clear about the background and necessity of antibiotic therapy (☞ Table 2.2). These reasons range from "convenience" or simple "reduction of symptoms" (e.g. in the case of diarrhea, otitis media, or bronchitis) to the treatment of the patient at risk of sepsis (☞ Table 2.2). Other local infections, in which elevated PCT levels could have been assumed based on clinical symptoms, often exhibit no PCT increase, since they are locally restricted. This is the case for appendicitis, cholecystitis, and tonsillitis, for example.

When using a higher limit value (e.g. at 0.5 ng/ml), however, e.g. in children, PCT is also able to distinguish significantly better between severe or potentially invasive bacterial infections and local infections or non-bacterial diseases than CRP. This was shown in a multi-center study in Spain (49) (☞ Sections 9.1. and 9.3.). High PCT levels should therefore always be considered cause for alarm, and, if necessary, be a reason for hospital admission.

Example for the practical use of PCT level measurement in outpatient cases

- A 25-year-old patient visits the doctor's office in November with symptoms of fever, cough, sniffles, expectoration (clear) and lassitude. The symptoms have persisted for three days. There is no acouophonic indication of regional ventilation problems, pronounced spasms, or collection of secreta. The PCT level of 0.15 ng/ml indicates that antibiotic treatment does not seem urgent at this time. The patient is scheduled for a follow-up in 2 days, or if symptoms worsen.

3. Biochemistry, pathophysiology

3.1. Procalcitonin (PCT), a soluble protein

Procalcitonin was first described as a sepsis-associated protein in 1993 (29). The protein consists of 116 amino acids and can be detected in the plasma during sepsis, infection, and severe inflammatory reactions (☞ Figure 1.1). The amino acid sequence is identical with that of the precursor protein of the hormone calcitonin; thus in its core area, it has the same amino acid sequence as calcitonin. Both proteins (PCT and calcitonin) stem from the same gene, but their induction is regulated differently. Procalcitonin induced by sepsis also originates in different cells than hormonally-active calcitonin, which is primarily synthesized by C-cells in the adrenal glands and partly by hormonally-active neuroendocrine cells in other organs.

Besides the complete prohormone (116 amino acids), different fragments of procalcitonin also appear in the plasma (☞ Figure 3.1). First, the plasma contains a form N-terminally truncated by two amino acids to 114 amino acids by the enzyme dipeptidyl peptidase IV (DPP IV), which may be biologically inactive for certain functions. Second, there are fragments of procalcitonin of varying length that include the calcitonin sequence with the corresponding N- or C-terminal end of the remainder of the molecule (55-60).

There are also two different types of procalcitonin (type I and type II). They differ only in the sequence of 8 C-terminal amino acids. They are produced in different tissues in different ratios (61). For the measurement of the PCT level in the blood, this difference, like that of the N-terminal truncation, is insignificant, since the available commercial assays detect both forms (62).

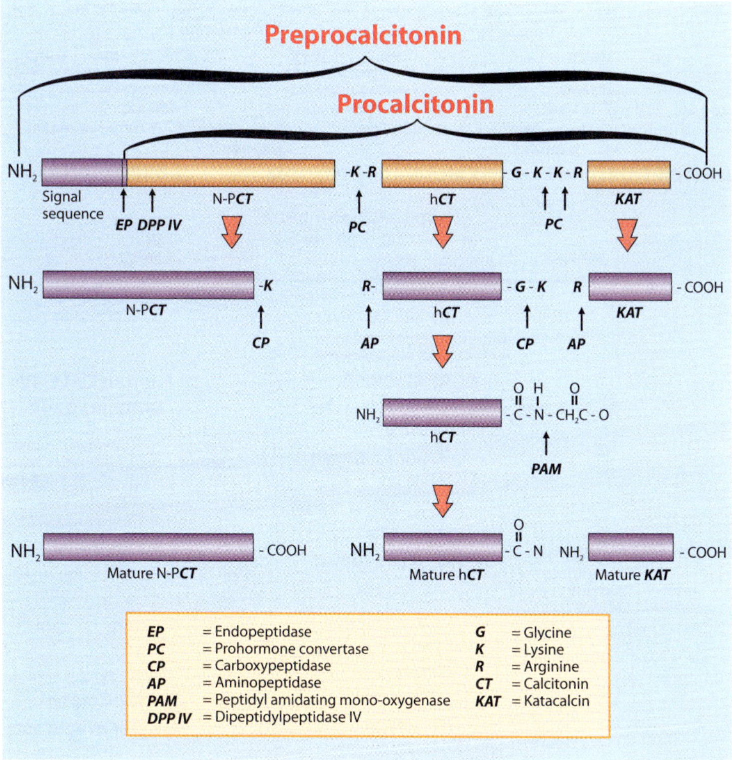

Figure 3.1: Cleavage of preprocalcitonin and procalcitonin by endopeptidases (modified according to (63) and (55)).

3.2. Genetics

Calcitonin and procalcitonin originate in CALC-I on chromosome 11 (11p, 15.4, EMBL access number X 15943) (64, 65). The proteins of this gene are an example of how a single gene can produce different proteins with different functions. This partly takes place due to a so-called "differential splicing" (gene products CGRP, PCT type I or II), and partly due to different processing of the finished protein (gene product calcitonin, PCT with 116 and 114 amino acids, as well as their fragments). "Differential splicing" means that a single gene can form different proteins due to different splicing of the messenger RNA (mRNA) (☞ Figure 3.2). The resulting proteins have partly different functions and – due to different induction mechanisms and induction conditions – appear in different concentrations in the individual cell types or organs. For example, the "calcitonin gene-related

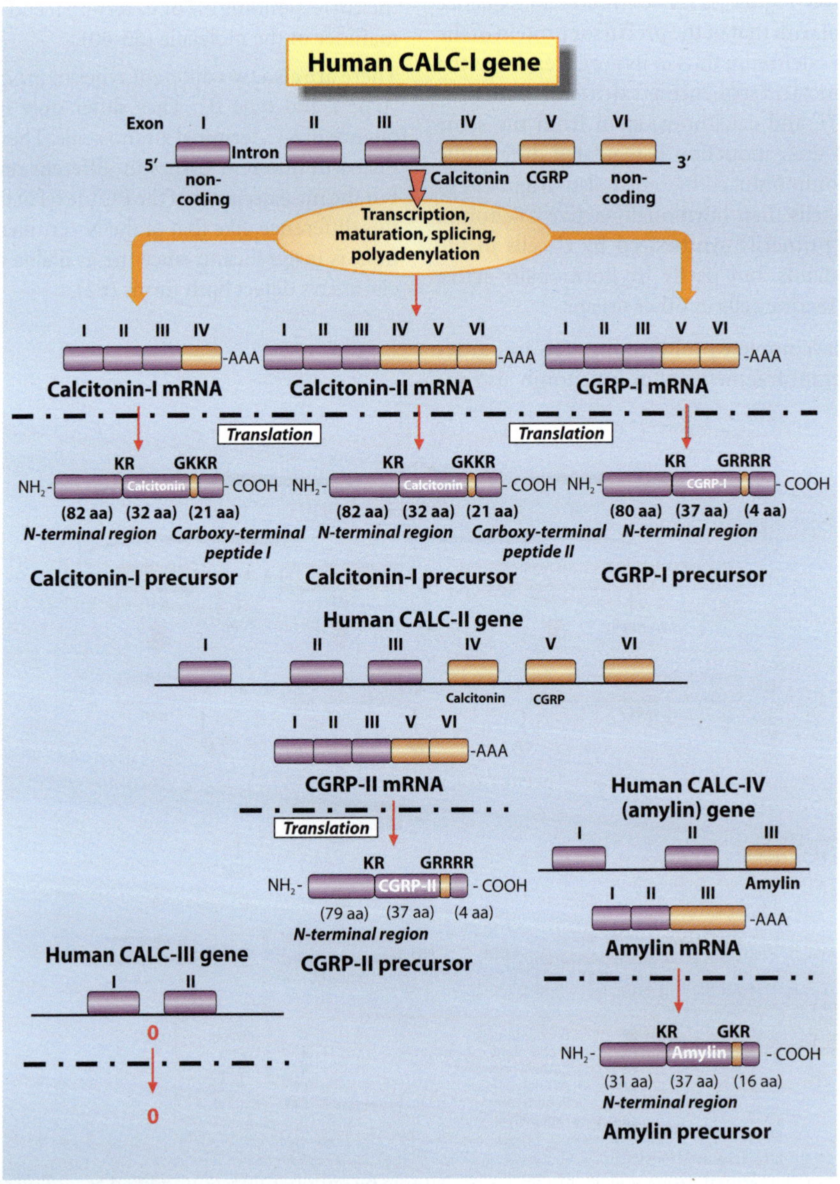

Figure 3.2: The gene family of the calcitonins (after (67)).

peptide" (CGRP) is a strongly vasodilatative substance, calcitonin is a hormone with influence on the calcium metabolism and functions in the central nervous system (pain processing), and procalcitonin is a substance that modulates the immune function. Whether the cleavage products of PCT have any function has not yet been examined (☞ overview (62) and (66)).

3.3. Mechanisms of induction and elimination of PCT

The induction of PCT is strictly regulated, requiring different steps for activation (☞ Figure 3.3). Unlike various cytokines, processes of adhesion and intercellular contacts (cell-to-cell communication) play a role, along with a time-dependent progression of cellular activation. The strict regulation of induction may be one reason for the high specificity of the marker, whose plasma concentration correlates well with the severity of the illness and/or degree of inflammatory activation.

Circulating monocytes also produce hardly any PCT after stimulation with high concentrations of endotoxins (68-70). Only adhering cells exhibit significant PCT production (☞ Figure 3.3, step 2). This persists only for a few hours (66). Only direct contact of adherent monocytary cells with parenchymatous cells – demonstrated to date only for adipocytes – leads to the production of PCT in these cells due to cell-to-cell interactions (☞ Figure 3.3 step 3) (61, 71, 72). Our knowledge of the induction mechanisms listed here is based on laboratory experiments (in vitro and/or ex vivo experiments). These provide our first explanations of why procalcitonin appears in nearly every tissue during sepsis. The liver – as a large and immunologically active organ and a filter for endotoxins –

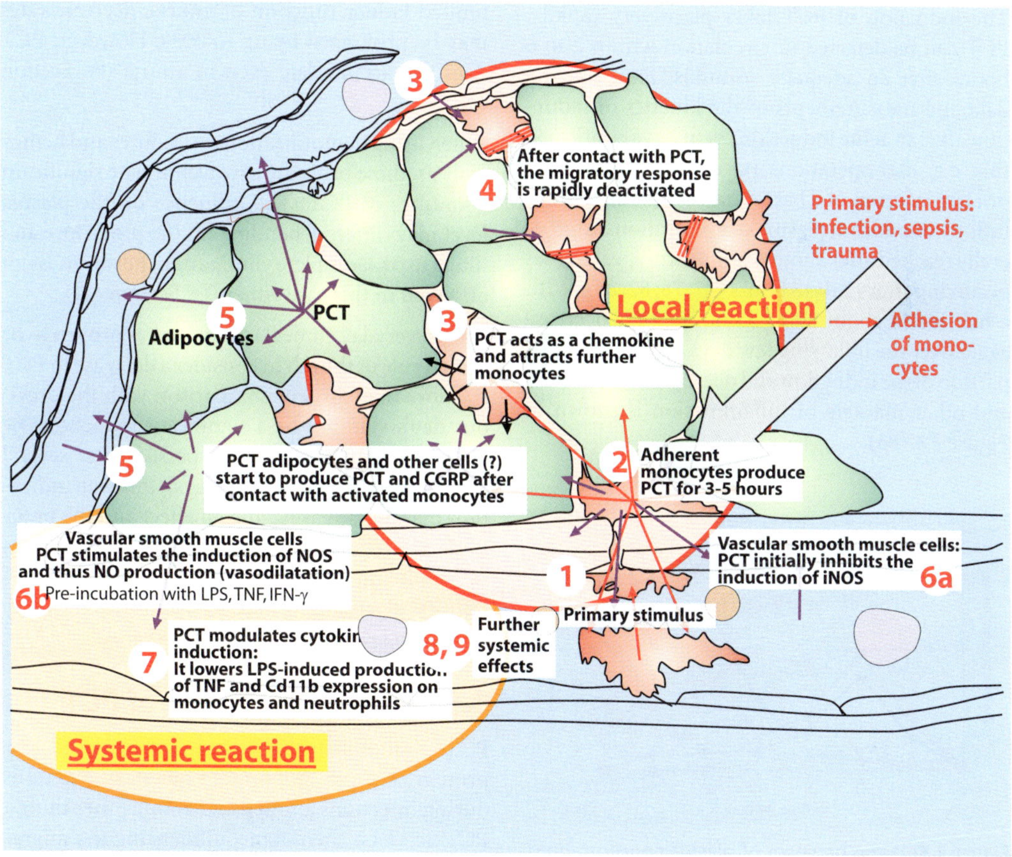

Figure 3.3: Induction and biological effects of PCT. In this diagram, the results of experimental examinations are summarized as a hypothetical model. The steps of activation are related both in time and in function. Numbers 1 through 8 in the diagram correspond to the explanations in Section 3.5. Modified after Linscheid.

also produced large quantities of PCT during sepsis (73-75). The necessity of cell-to-cell interaction as a prerequisite for induction also explains why only very little PCT can be detected in circulation in local infections, while sepsis or endotoxin injection can reliably produce high concentrations (66). Even the temporary formation of PCT after extended operations or severe tissue trauma can be explained in this manner.

Systemically, not only after injection with endotoxin but also after injection with proinflammatory cytokines, we can observe the formation of PCT (73, 76-81).

3.4. Time behavior of induction and elimination

▶ Experimental data on induction kinetics

The induction of PCT takes place very rapidly. PCT can be detected in circulation within 2 to 6 hours after an adequate stimulus. Experimental data and measurements of the kinetics of induction after an acute induction event have confirmed this (e.g. after operations, injection of endotoxins, or after infusion of a bacterially contaminated solution). Significant plasma concentrations are generally reached after about 6 hours, with peak values occurring after 12 to 48 hours (77, 78, 82, 83). With a half-life of about 20 to 35 hours, they decrease again over the following few days (77, 79). A comparison of the induction and decrease times of PCT and other markers of inflammation is shown in Figure 3.4 (83).

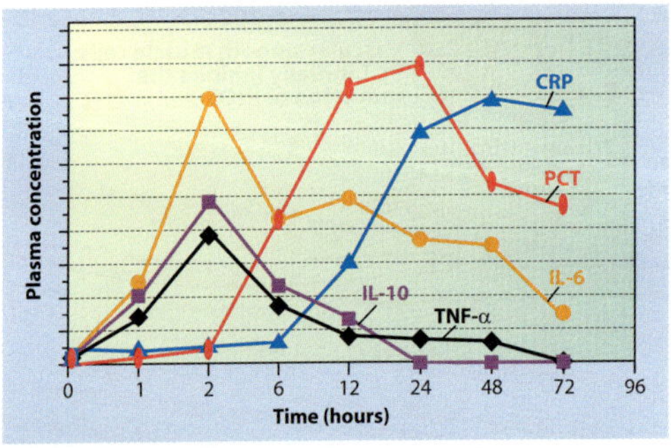

Figure 3.4: Time behavior of plasma concentrations of procalcitonin, C-reactive protein, and cytokines after operative trauma (thoracic surgery). Schematic representation (83).

▶ The clinically observed half-life

The clinically observed behavior of the concentration of a plasma protein – and thus the clinically observed elimination half-life – depends essentially on the difference between new production and decomposition or elimination of the corresponding substance. The "decrease rate" (plasma disappearance rate) thus measured should not be confused with the biological half-life of the protein. After acute one-time induction, the clinically observed half-life of PCT is about 20 to 24 hours, in some cases a little longer (77-79). In critically ill patients in intensive care, measurement of the time behavior of PCT concentrations can also be used to determine clinical decrease rates after an induction event of limited duration. In this case, the values – possibly due to longer production of the substance – are only slightly longer than one day, averaging between 25 and 30 hours (27, 28, 84). In the case of limited kidney function or anuria, decrease rates may be prolonged by up to 30%. However, PCT does not accumulate even in anuria (☞ Section 8.4.).

When using hemofiltration procedures and hemodialysis, these procedures can eliminate significant quantities of PCT. The influence on the plasma level may differ, depending on the procedure and filters used. Complete elimination, however, is not observed in this case either (☞ Section 8.4).

In the everyday clinical routine, it has proven to be a good rule of thumb to consider a decrease in PCT by more than 30% in comparison with the previous day's value to be a significant reduction (☞ Figure 2.5). If this tendency persists over several days (generally at least three days), this is an indication that therapy is having an effect and the prognosis is favorable. PCT thus reacts kinetically significantly more quickly than C-reactive protein – both in terms of its formation and in terms of decay of plasma levels.

3.5. Biological effects of PCT

PCT is a modulator of the immune response. The protein performs important regulatory functions during infections and sepsis. Among other things, PCT acts as a chemokine, influencing the migratory response of monocytary cells (85). PCT also modulates the induction of proinflammatory cytokines. These effects, however, are slight. They may be mediated by influence of the cAMP system (85, 88-90). Moreover – depending on the activation of the cells – the induction of inducible NO-synthase, responsible for the regulation of vascular dilation during infection and sepsis, is either inhibited or stimulated (86, 87). PCT inhibits the stimulation of the CGRP-1 receptor by CGRP and is simultaneously a partial agonist of this receptor and of the adrenomedullin-1 (AMY-1) receptor (365). It is speculated that the N-terminal proteolytic cleavage of PCT by dipeptidyl peptidase IV (DP IV) leads to the inactivation of biological function (for example of chemotaxis) (55).

Biological effects of PCT:

- Effect as chemokine (time-dependent)
- Modulation of release of proinflammatory cytokines
- Modulation of vascular contraction (iNOS induction) (time-dependent)
- Inhibition of the effects of CGRP and partial agonist of the CGRP-1 and AMY-1 receptors
- Influence on mortality in animal experimental model
- Influence on circulation and kidney function in animal experimental model

Experimentally, in bacterial shock in hamsters subject to neutralization of PCT, an increased survival rate can be observed, while administration of PCT leads to an increase in mortality (91, 92) (☞ Figure 3.5). In pigs, the protective effect of PCT neutralization can also be seen on the progression of endotoxin shock: when PCT is neutralized, the average arterial pressure and the pH value of the blood decreased less sharply, while the increase in creatinine values was lessened (93, 94). Antibodies against PCT have not yet been used for therapeutic purposes in humans.

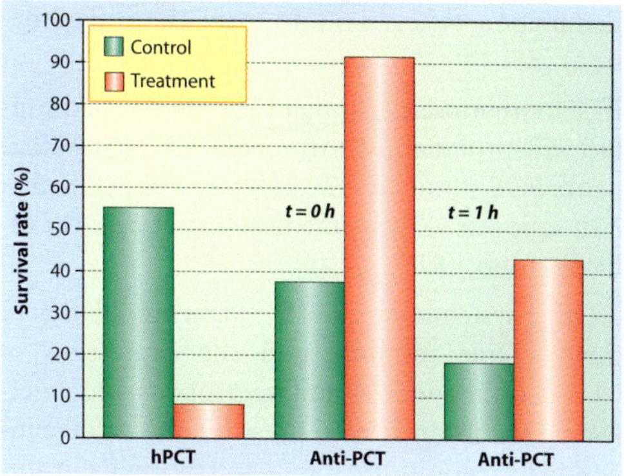

Figure 3.5: Influence of procalcitonin on bacterial shock in hamsters: Administration of human PCT leads to increased mortality (group hPCT), while anti-PCT effective antibodies have a protective effect. The protective effect can be seen both in prophylactic administration (Anti-PCT group on the left) and in therapeutic application (Anti-PCT group right) (after (91)).

This data, together with the complex mechanisms of induction, can be used to formulate a hypothetical model of the induction and immunological effects of PCT (☞ Figure 3.3):

▶ Model of a biological effect of PCT

1. A primary stimulus (e.g. a local or systemic infection, tissue trauma, sepsis) leads to the expression of adhesion molecules and thus to the adherence of monocytes (☞ step 1, Figure 3.3).

2. These start with the production of PCT, which lasts about 3 to 5 hours and then ends (66, 95, 96) (☞ step 2, Figure 3.3).

3. The local release of PCT acts as a chemokine and attracts additional activated monocytes, which penetrate the tissue (☞ steps 2 and 4, Figure 3.3).

4. The migratory reaction triggered by PCT is time-dependent and is deactivated after a few hours by the presence of PCT. The cells thus remain at the site of the inflammation (85).

5. Adipocytes (and possibly other parenchymatous cells, as well), after direct contact with activated monocytes, start production of PCT and CGRP (☞ step 3, Figure 3.3) (66).

6. The biochemical effects of PCT are time-dependent on the activation state of the target cells (☞ steps 5 through 8): in native smooth muscle cells of the endothelium, PCT inhibits the induction of inducible NO-synthase (iNOS), an enzyme responsible for NO-mediated vascular dilation during in-

flammation (effect remote from the inflammation) (86).

In smooth muscle cells that have already had contact with proinflammatory mediators, on the other hand, PCT stimulates the induction of iNOS, that is, it supports vascular dilation (effect near the inflammation) (87).

7. Other systemic effects of PCT are: modulation of the cytokine response and the expression of CD11b on monocytes and neutrophils and an effect on the mean arterial pressure, the cardiac index, pH, creatinine clearance and mortality in animal models of endotoxin shock (80, 91, 93, 97, 98). As a result, a modification of function may possibly occur through proteolytic cleavage of the protein from 116 to 114 amino acids by the enzyme DP IV (termination of the chemotactic effect?).

In addition to the effects described, there is also an inhibition of stimulation of CGRP-1 receptors by CGRP in the presence of CGRP. PCT is also a partial agonist of the adrenomedullin-1 and CGRP-1 receptors (365).

Other in vitro studies show that, after stimulation by IL-1β or endotoxin, differentiated adipocytes produce PCT, while interferon-γ inhibits this process. This is possibly another reason why PCT is expressed particularly in bacterial infections but not in viral infection (384).

During local infections, the effects of PCT listed may be advantageous. PCT regulates the collection of monocytes for a limited time and modulates vascular dilation. This is stimulated at the site of the inflammation but inhibited in the surrounding region. If there is already a systemic inflammatory response, the effects of PCT must rather be seen as unfavorable (☞ animal experiments, Figure 3.5).

4. Laboratory chemistry

4.1. Methods of PCT level measurement

There are various immunoassays available, including automated ones, for the quantitative or semi-quantitative measurement of procalcitonin. Depending on the method, measurement is possible in serum or plasma, and depending on the assay selected, 20 to 200 µl samples are needed. The time until a PCT result is available is 19 minutes to 2.5 hours after the start of the test. The most important criterion for the selection of the measurement method is the clinical question asked (e.g. highly sensitive measurement for antibiotic monitoring, small sample volume in pediatrics). It must be noted that not every measurement procedure can measure the lower reference range (concentrations <0.1 ng/ml) with sufficient accuracy. Automated PCT measurement methods, with analytical assay sensitivities of as little as 0.02 ng/ml, have the lowest detection limits as well as outstanding precision.

The following measurement methods are available:

- Semi-quantitative using solid-phase-coupled immune diffusion (e.g. PCT-Q test).
- Diverse quantitative procedures:
    - Manual, semiautomated, or automated measurement procedures for different laboratory systems.

Information about assay-specific characteristics (assay sensitivity, sample preparation) as well as about measurement methods can be found in the device-specific technical information provided by the specific manufacturer and on www.procalcitonin.com.

4.2. Stability and half-life in vitro, preanalytical factors

▶ Stability in the blood sample

In blood samples, in contrast to most cytokines, PCT is very stable. At room temperature, the PCT plasma concentration decreases by only about 12% in the 24 hours after samples are taken, and by only about 6% when stored at 4°C (26). Thus PCT can be sampled together with other serum and plasma samples in the context of a routine blood draw and sent to the laboratory, with no need for special storage.

Samples should only be cooled or frozen immediately until level measurement in case of longer storage or transport times, or if study parameters do not allow for any external influence on samples.

Freezing of samples does not significantly change the plasma or serum concentrations. It is also of slight significance which anticoagulant is used, or whether plasma or serum, arterial or venous samples are used for the measurement. However, a standardized sample technique, anticoagulant, and storage should be agreed upon within a laboratory association and hospital, as well as sample transport (26).

4.3. Normal values and reference ranges of PCT

In healthy subjects, the plasma level of PCT is below 0.05 ng/ml. In older patients and patients with different pre-existing conditions, in less than 10% of cases a slightly higher PCT level has been measured (up to above 0.1 ng/ml, but usually under 0.3 ng/ml) (48). The threshold for diagnosis of sepsis, on the other hand, is significantly higher, at 0.5 ng/ml (500 pg/ml). This concentration range is reliably detected by all current measurement procedures.

Procalcitonin reacts very dynamically to bacterial inflammatory illnesses. Concentrations of more than 1000 ng/ml have been measured in individual cases. Such concentrations, however, are very rare; levels in severe sepsis or septic shock are more frequently in a range from 5 to 500 ng/ml (☞ Figure 1.2).

The reference ranges for important indications, with guidelines for interpretation, are given in Table 2.1 and Figure 2.4.

5. PCT as a marker of infection and sepsis: an evidence-based collection of data

5.1. Differential diagnosis of bacterial infections: SIRS and sepsis

Numerous studies support the high diagnostic reliability of PCT for the diagnosis of sepsis and for severe bacterial infections. If PCT induction is not exhibited despite a clinically observable systemic inflammatory response, non-bacterial causes of the illness are probable. Depending on the clinical situation and individual existing diseases, these may be viral infections, autoimmune diseases, or a "SIRS" of a different origin (☞ Table 5.1). In individual cases, a local bacterial infection may be present, if the systemic inflammatory symptoms are still not clearly expressed and have not yet led to the induction of PCT. A more detailed picture of the indications in different specializations can be found in the following Chapters 6. through 8..

In patients with "SIRS" or uncomplicated sepsis (sepsis without organ dysfunction), the limits of the PCT levels measured may sometimes be somewhat fluid. For only slightly elevated PCT concentrations, therefore, the measured values should be carefully interpreted with reference to the clinical context. For numerous illnesses, however, it has been possible to evaluate the diagnostic significance of PCT very precisely. These illnesses are listed below, with references to the corresponding studies and uses.

Diagnosis	Cut-off	Sensitivity Specificity	PCT (ng/ml) (ave., average)	Number of patients	Literature
Acute meningitis: viral versus bacterial infection (children)	>0.5 µg/l	94% 100%	(ave., range) 0.32 (0-1.7) 54.5 (4.8-110)	41 18	(99)
Autoimmune diseases: no infection versus bacterial infection	>0.5 g/l	100% 84%	<0.5 1.9 ± 1.19	42 16	(100)
Kidney transplantation: acute rejection infection	>0.5 µg/l	87% 70%	- -	13 17	(37)
Pneumonia: bacterial atypical agent	- -	- -	(ave., range) 1.41 (0.05-65) 0.05 (0.05-7.5	27 9	(101)
Pneumonia: bacterial viral agent	2 ng/ml	63% 96%	(ave., range) 2.7 (0.6-91) 0.63 (0.01-4.38)	43 29	(102)
Infections in children invasive local	0.9 ng/ml	93% 78%	(ave., SD) 27.5 ± 70 0.32 ± 0.32	64 27	(103)
Pancreatitis, edematous: sterile necroses infected necroses	>1.8 µg/l	94% 91%	- -	18 14 18	(104)
Patients in intensive care: no infection with infection	>0.6 µg/l	67% 61%	0.5 (median) 2.5 (median)	79 111	(105)

Table 5.1: Serum/plasma concentrations of procalcitonin and its sensitivity and specificity values for different cut-off values for the diagnosis of illnesses with bacterial and non-bacterial causes.

Viral infections

In viral illnesses, PCT values are generally not increased or are increased only slightly, while in sepsis due to bacterial causes, PCT values of over 0.5 ng/ml to over 2 ng/ml are often observed. PCT can therefore contribute – for example in cases of nonspecific clinical symptoms and a corresponding suspicion of illness – to distinguishing between viral and bacterial infections (☞ Table 5.1, Sections 7.5. and 9.3.).

There are examinations for viral and bacterial meningitis (34, 99, 106-109), infections of the respiratory tract (110-112), as well as case descriptions of systemic viral infections (HIV, SARS) (113-114). See also Section 9.3. (differential diagnoses between viral and bacterial infections in children).

Autoimmune diseases

Only in exceptional cases is there any significant induction of PCT in autoimmune diseases. Particularly in autoimmune diseases with significant systemic inflammatory activation or in severe vasculitis ("Anti-neutrophile cytoplasmatic antibody positive vasculitis", or ANCA, Wegener's Disease, Still's Disease, or Kawasaki Syndrome) can PCT values of over 0.5 ng/ml or, even more rarely, of over 1 ng/ml, be seen. PCT values of over 5 ng/ml have been observed in Kawasaki Syndrome and Still's Disease (115-117). In other autoimmune disease (Crohn's Disease, ulcerative colitis, rheumatoid arthritis, systemic erythmatic lupus, systemic sclerodermia, sarcoidosis, or thyroiditis, etc.), PCT – in contrast with other markers of inflammation (e.g. CRP or IL-6) – is not significantly induced.

A differentiation of severe bacterial infection is possible with PCT even in patients with inflammatory symptoms due to autoimmune diseases (☞ Figure 5.1). See also Section 7.7 on this topic.

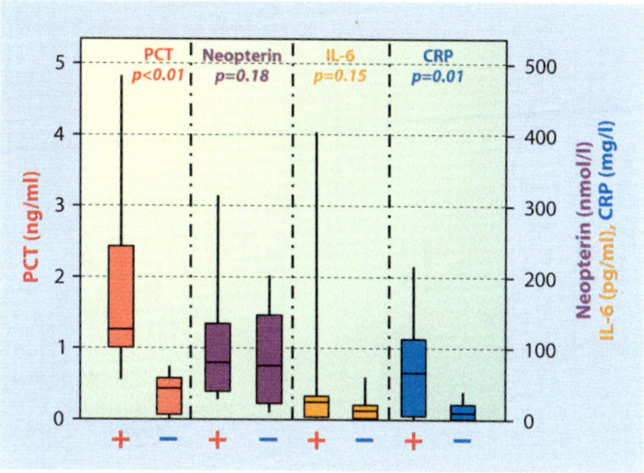

Figure 5.1: Serum concentrations of PCT, neopterin, IL-6, and CRP in 11 patients with antibody-associated vasculitis during 16 episodes of systemic infection, in comparison with an infection-free interval of 4 to 6 weeks, or after therapy (p, Wilcoxon test) (100).

Organ transplantation and rejection reaction

An acute rejection reaction after organ transplantation generally induces no PCT. The marker can therefore distinguish between sepsis and inflammatory symptoms due to rejection reactions in these patients (☞ Figure 5.2).

The therapy is entirely different in the two cases. While in one case immunosuppression must be reduced and antibiotic therapy reinforced, in the other case more extensive immune suppression is required. In exceptional cases, PCT levels can also be elevated due to severe organ damage or organ necrosis (e.g. due to lack of perfusion). Extensive specifications for PCT level measurement after heart, liver, and kidney transplants can be found in Section 8.3..

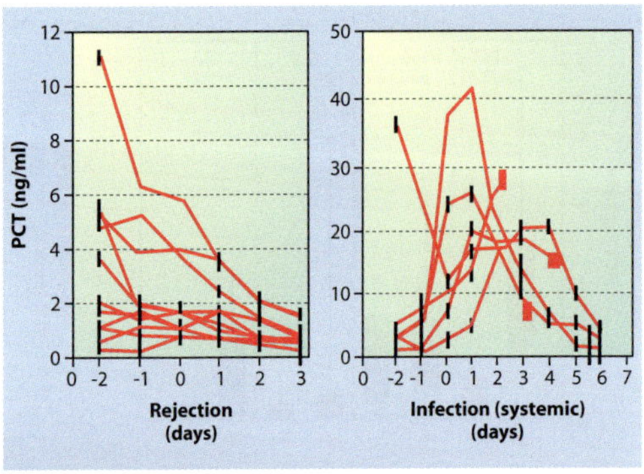

Figure 5.2: Behavior of plasma concentration of PCT after liver transplantation in patients with rejection reactions (left) or systemic infection (right). + = non-survival. An increase in PCT is easy to see during sepsis (0, day of diagnosis) (40).

▶ Local infections and "severe infections"

PCT also distinguishes between local bacterial infections and infections clinically described as "severe infections" – even though these terms are not used uniformly. "Severe infections" are generally potentially life-threatening, or they trigger systemic activation of the immune system. Different studies support the superiority of PCT over CRP in such cases (☞ Figure 5.3a and 5.3b) (49, 118). If PCT levels are elevated or increasing, therefore, it is always necessary to arrange for an (antibiotic) therapy or hospitalization, while for normal or very low PCT levels it is at least possible to consider avoiding them.

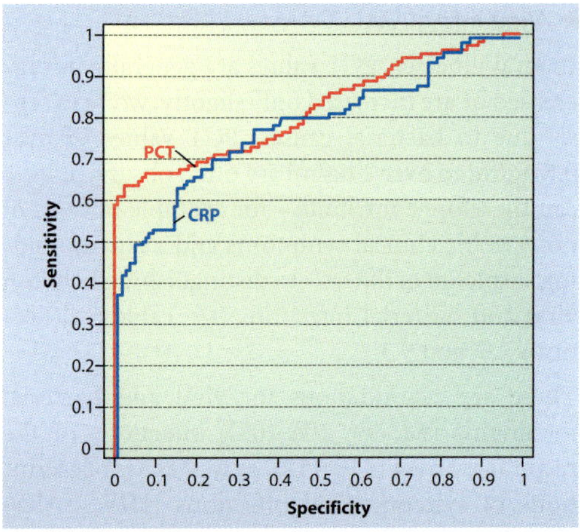

a

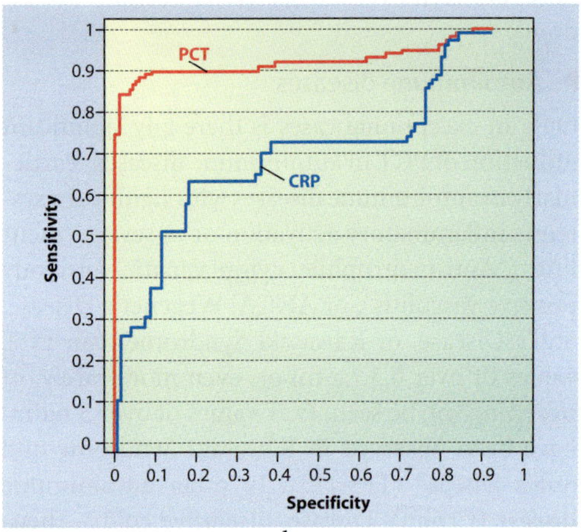

b

Figures 5.3a+b: Procalcitonin (PCT) and C-reactive protein (CRP) in children with fever in pediatric emergency admissions. The figure shows the ROC diagram of sensitivity and specificity of both measured values for the differential diagnosis of viral infection and less-invasive bacterial infections (☞ Figure 5.3a, left) and of less-invasive versus potentially invasive bacterial infections (☞ Figure 5.3b, right). In this important distinction, PCT is the only marker examined to differ with high sensitivity and specificity in patients with severe or potentially invasive infections. The area under the curve on the left is 0.82 for PCT and 0.78 for CRP, and on the right 0.95 for PCT and 0.81 for CRP (49).

▶ "SIRS" and "sepsis"

PCT is one of the best markers available for the clinical routine diagnosis of sepsis. Meta-analyses have demonstrated the superiority of this marker over the classical infection marker CRP (41, 42) (☞ Figure 5.4 and Figure 5.5).

A reliable distinction between "SIRS" and "sepsis", however, is not always possible based on PCT data alone. This has been shown in various studies and a meta-analysis (☞ Table 5.2) (43). There could be different reasons for this observation. The induction trigger for PCT is probably still weak for bacterially induced "sepsis". However, in that case there is generally no danger to the patient of organ dysfunction. Conversely, there are numerous situations in which PCT can be induced to a slight extent by a non-bacterial ("nonspecific") inflammatory reaction. Moreover, the primary goal of most studies was not to differentiate between "SIRS" and "sepsis". The response to this question is thus "blurry", for example because known causes for a non-bacterial induction of PCT were not prospectively excluded (e.g. postoperative or post-traumatic patients). The type and severity of bacterial infection was also not sufficiently differentiated in most studies. Studies or meta-analyses including patients with a highly severe sepsis in the evaluation, however, show the high diagnostic reliability of PCT (13, 41, 42).

▶ Progression of infection and sepsis towards "severe sepsis"

For the diagnosis of a "severe sepsis" or "septic shock," PCT has a very high predictive value (☞ Section 5.3). This is due to the fact that PCT reacts reliably in these illnesses, and serum levels frequently exceed more than 2 ng/ml. For values of over 10 ng/ml, the diagnosis of a "severe sepsis" or "septic shock" is very probable (☞ Table 5.3, Figure 1.4). PCT is therefore approved in the United States for use on the first day of intensive care with the indication of the diagnosis of a progression towards "severe sepsis" or "septic shock" (☞ Section 1.4.).

Diagnosis	n	PCT (ng/ml)	Sensitivity (%)	Specificity (%)	Literature
Sepsis	190	0,6	68	61	(105)
Sepsis	101	1	89	94	(13)
Sepsis	101	2	65	70	(119)
Septic shock	60	5	88	67	(120)
Sepsis	78	1.1	97	78	(33)
SIRS/sepsis	101	1.2	63	87	(6)
Sepsis in pancreatitis	61	1.8	95	88	(104)
Fever or septic shock	208	0.8	68	48	(121)

Table 5.2: Sensitivity and specificity of PCT in the differentiation of SIRS and sepsis for different cut-off values. N = the number of patients examined, PCT = procalcitonin, SIRS = Systemic inflammatory response syndrome.

SIRS Median (*), range Mean (+), SD	Sepsis	Severe sepsis	Septic shock	Number of patients	Literature
- -	2.4 ± 0.5 (+)	37 ± 16	45 ± 22	145	(123)
0.6 ± 2.2$^+$	6.6 ± 22.5	- -	35 ± 68	337	(124)
1.3 ± 0.2$^+$	2.0 ± 0	8.7 ± 2.5	39 ± 5,9	100	(125)
<0.5 ng/ml*	0.8 ng/ml	- -	4.3 ng/ml	190	(105)
3.8 ± 6.9$^+$	1.3 ± 2.7	9.1 ± 18.2	38 ± 59	101	(119)
3.0 (0.7-29.5)*	- -	19.1 (2.8-351)	16.8 (0.9-351) *"all septic patients"*	33	(126)
0.5 ± 0.2$^+$ (roughly)	2 ± 2 (roughly)	18 ± 10 (roughly)	20 ± 10 (roughly)	101	(13)
0.38* (0.16-0.93 quartile)	3.0 (1.48-15.3)	5.58 (1.84-32.9)	13.1 (6.1-42.2)	101	(6)
0.6 (0-5.3)*	3.5 (0.4-6.7)	6.2 (2.2-85)	21.3 (1.2-654)	78	(33)

Table 5.3: Serum and plasma concentrations of PCT for different severities of Systemic Inflammatory Response Syndrome and sepsis.

▶ The diagnostic limit can be used for "risk evaluation"

The limit value and thus the diagnostic reliability for a clinical decision selected in an individual case is the decision of the physician, depending on the clinical conditions themselves (existing disease in the patient, clinical situation, symptoms) (☞ "Special indications for PCT level measurement").

It must always be taken into consideration that the interpretation of PCT is an evaluation of risks and probabilities (☞ Figure 1.6). The use of pure cut-off values can therefore lead to misinterpretation in some cases. The probability of a sepsis, severe sepsis, or septic shock increases with higher PCT levels, while low PCT values make these diagnoses increasingly improbable.

> PCT is a marker of sepsis, that is, a marker of infection and inflammation. High levels are an indication of increasingly high risk of the presence of sepsis, severe sepsis, or septic shock.

If a limit value is still desirable for the diagnosis, a concentration of 0.5 ng/ml can be seen as a guideline for the diagnosis of sepsis, distinguishing between "SIRS" and "sepsis," or between an "uncomplicated" or "complicated" or "severe" infection. In local infections (e.g. COPD), on the other hand, the PCT level generally stays in a range far below this level (e.g. under 0.25 ng/ml to under 0.1 ng/ml).

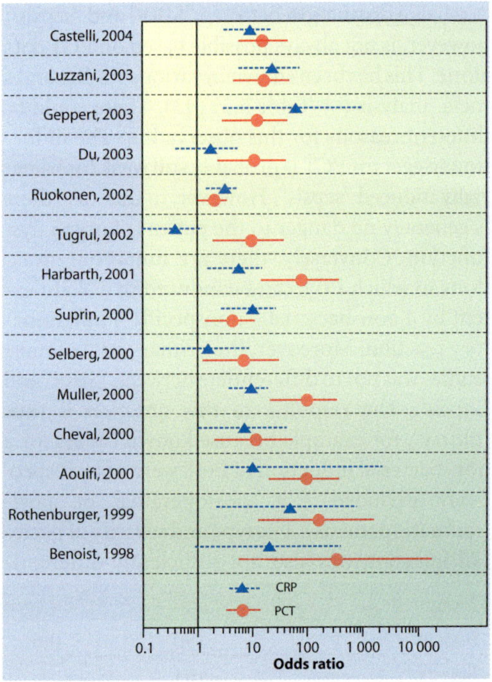

Figure 5.4: Odds Ratio (OR) of the diagnostic precision of a diagnosis of infection or sepsis, severe sepsis, and septic shock in comparison with "SIRS" without septic (bacterial) cause, for PCT and CRP. 15 studies were involved in the calculation in comparison with CRP. The global OR for PCT was 12.16. That means that the risk of measuring positive PCT (>0.5 ng/ml) in patients with bacterial infections, sepsis, severe sepsis, or septic shock is 12 times higher than in patients without bacterial infection. The value of the OR for CRP, on the other hand, is only 5.75. If studies are considered that only measured PCT (without comparison with CRP) (n=25 studies), the OR for PCT is even higher, at 14.9 (95% CI 7.1:30.3) for CRP 5.4 (95% CI 3.2:9.2) (42).

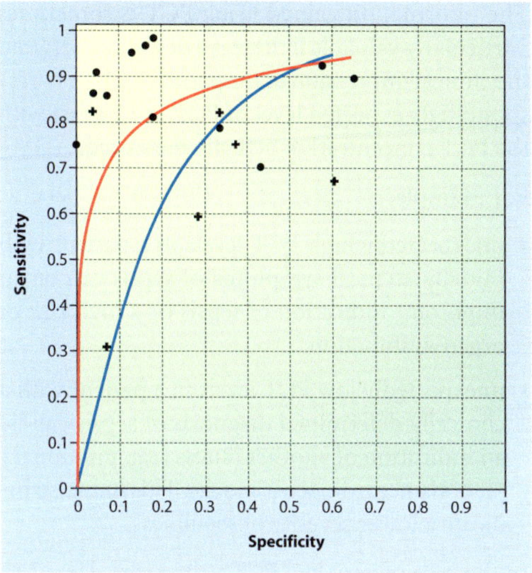

Figure 5.5: Total ROC diagram of a meta-analysis of PCT (red line) and CRP (blue line) for the differential diagnosis of bacterial infection in patients with signs of inflammation, in comparison with non-bacterial causes of an inflammatory response. 12 studies were included in the meta-analysis. Each point represents a study included in the analysis (41).

5.2. PCT as a marker of the progression of infection to sepsis, severe sepsis and septic shock

PCT reflects the progression of a local infection or "sepsis only" (sepsis without organ dysfunction) to "severe sepsis" or "septic shock" particularly well (☞ Table 5.3, Figures 1.4 and 2.1). These forms of disease are characterized by severe complications and an increasingly mortality risk.

This indication largely corresponds to the approval indication for PCT in the United States by the FDA (Food and Drug Administration) (☞ Section 1.4.).

The progression of sepsis to severe sepsis is generally characterized by a marked increase in PCT.

With increasing PCT levels, therefore, the probability rises that a patient has sepsis, severe sepsis, or septic shock. Already at levels over 0.5 ng/ml – depending on the study – this probability may be over 63% and even as high as 97% (6, 33). In a meta-analysis, the odds ratio for the diagnosis of a severe infection (that is, in this context, an infection with systemic inflammatory response) was over 14.6 for PCT and only 5.4 for CRP (☞ Figure 5.4) (42). For PCT levels above 10 ng/ml, the diagnosis is nearly certain, as long as no other known factors can explain the increased PCT (122).

The reliability of the diagnosis of sepsis can be improved by simultaneous PCT level measurement along with evaluation of clinical data and measurement of conventional values.

In everyday clinical practice, it is of extreme importance to detect the progression of an infection or sepsis to severe sepsis and septic shock quickly and reliably, since the rate of mortality increases rapidly with increasing organ dysfunction (☞ Figure 1.3).

The progression of sepsis to severe sepsis is associated with an increase in mortality.

The progression of an infection or sepsis to severe forms of the disease must therefore be prevented early by the timely intervention of all available means. These primarily include adequate antibiotic therapy, if necessary a timely and decisive focal surgery, and measures to prevent an increase in organ dysfunction, since these are associated with increased mortality. This includes, among other things, an optimization of perfusion as well as specific and adjuvant measures (127).

When determining the progression of an infection towards sepsis, severe sepsis, and septic shock, PCT is superior to numerous other markers – particularly CRP. The reliability of the clinical diagnosis can also be improved with simultaneous use of PCT (☞ Figure 2.2) (33).

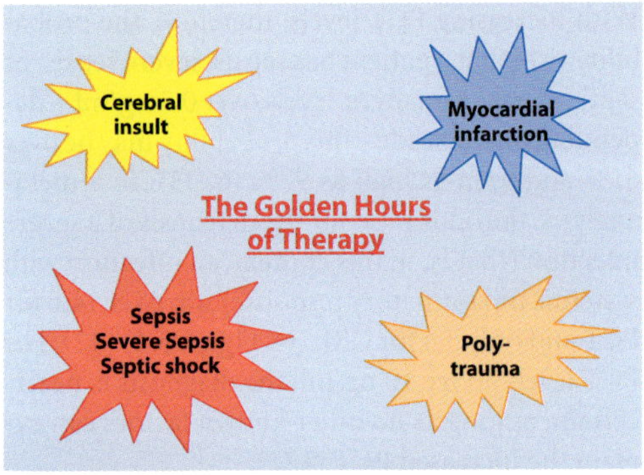

Figure 5.6: The "golden hours" of early therapy to improve the probability of survival and to avoid consequent damage also apply to the treatment of sepsis.

Mistakes in therapy made at an earlier point – if the advance stages of severe sepsis have been entered – are nearly impossible to compensate, even with difficult and cost-intensive treatment (☞ Figure 1.3) (30, 32, 128).

Thus the performance and time behavior of corresponding diagnostic and therapeutic measures should be checked and optimized using quality control measures in the individual departments or hospitals (☞ http://www.sepsis-benchmark.com, http://www.qmits-projekt.de).

The rules describing the "golden hours" of a speedy commencement of therapy not only apply to myocardial infarct, cerebral insult, and polytrauma, but also in patients with sepsis and severe sepsis (☞ Figure 5.6).

5.3. Interpretation of PCT in the clinical context

PCT is an indirect marker of sepsis and systemic inflammation. The induction of PCT is usually the consequence of a severe bacterial infection. It depends on the type and severity of the systemic inflammatory response. Moreover, there are situations in which PCT can be induced without the presence of a bacterial infection. PCT levels must therefore always be interpreted in the clinical context.

PCT levels must always be interpreted in the clinical context.

The information gained using PCT is sometimes particularly valuable if there is a deviation between the clinical impression of the patient and the correspondingly expected level of PCT in contrast with the PCT concentration actually measured.

For example,

- unexpectedly high PCT levels in a patient with initially atypical symptoms of sepsis can be an important indication of sepsis or a high risk of organ dysfunction.
- unexpectedly low PCT levels in a patient with a clinically determined diagnosis of sepsis can be an indication of another illness (e.g. pulmonary embolism, cardiogenic shock). This may also indicate a lower severity of the illness.

In the case of very low PCT values, the danger to the patient of sepsis or organ failure is less probable. Except from very fulminant conditions, there is usually time to confirm the diagnosis with no immediate danger to the patient due to sepsis.

In the case of high PCT levels, however, the prescription of a broadly-effective antibiotic should be started early and generously (calculated antibiotic therapy) and sepsis treatment begun immediately according to the guidelines for sepsis therapy. This includes an urgent search for the focus and/or surgery on such a focus. If necessary, it is recommended that the levels be checked after 6 to 12 hours.

In clinical practice, a discrepancy between the clinical condition of the patient and the PCT level measured can provide important information.

5.4. PCT: a marker of infection or of inflammation?

It is often asked whether PCT is a marker of infection or of inflammation. PCT is a marker which "indirectly" indicates the reaction of the body to an infection – in contrast to microbiological "direct" evidence of agents or their components (microbiological growth, detection of antigen, DNA analysis).

PCT is a marker of the organism's "host response" to a bacterial infection. It is therefore an "indirect" marker of infection.

The induction of PCT thus requires multiple conditions:

- On the one hand, the triggering stimulus, whether local or systemic, as the trigger of the host response (usually a bacterial infection or a tissue trauma),
- On the other hand, the activation of the immune response of the organism (systemic inflammatory response, transmitted e.g. by the adherence of monocytary cells, interaction of those cells with the tissue). There is a smooth transition between locally observed effects and a systematically demonstrable inflammatory response.
- And thirdly, a certain strength of this inflammatory reaction.

> PCT is generally induced by systemic inflammatory responses occurring as a consequence of bacterial infection.

Systemically effective inflammatory reactions with consequent damage to organ function are a significant cause of increased mortality in patients with infections. PCT level measurement as an indicator of a bacterially induced systemic inflammatory response is therefore a clinically practical measure, since PCT provides precisely this information (☞ Figure 1.3 and 1.4).

> The cause of increased mortality in patients with bacterial infections is usually not locally destructive processes of infection, but the impairment of organ function as a consequence of the systemic inflammatory response.

Laboratory chemical values which merely describe the presence of an infection without permitting quantitative description of the systemic inflammatory response thus include only one (limited) dimension of bacterial infectious disease in critically ill patients. In comparison with PCT, they have a weaker information content, since the "second dimension" (the severity of the illness) is missing. These markers include sTREM-1 (soluble triggering receptor expressed on myeloid cells), MBL (mannan-binding lectin), to a certain extent LBP (lipopolysaccharide-binding protein), and CRP (C-reactive protein) (379). These markers can therefore not be considered "sepsis markers" on their own.

▶ How strongly are the two dimensions of "infection and inflammation" involved in the induction of PCT?

To distinguish the role infection plays in contrast to the severity of the disease (organ dysfunction) in the induction of PCT, a study by Castelli et al. examined PCT and CRP levels in patients with and without infection at a comparable severity of organ dysfunction (measured with the SOFA score) (☞ Figure 5.7 and Figure 5.8) (6).

It can be seen that for a comparable severity of organ dysfunction, PCT levels in patients with simultaneous infection were higher on average than in patients without infection. This indicates that PCT is a relatively "infection-specific" marker. For CRP, on the other hand, the dependency on the severity of organ dysfunction in patients with and without infections was low, and levels were already elevated in patients without organ dysfunction. These data confirm the relatively nonspecific induction of CRP and the low correlation of CRP with the severity of the illness (6). The low correlation of CRP with the severity of illness and organ dysfunction is shown by several studies (6, 12, 49, 108, 134, 367).

> CRP – in contrast with PCT – is not a reliable marker of either infection or inflammation in critically ill patients.

Different studies agree that PCT has a higher sensitivity and specificity than CRP in terms of diagnosing sepsis, severe sepsis, or septic shock (☞ Figures 4.5 and 5.5, Table 5.4) (41, 42).

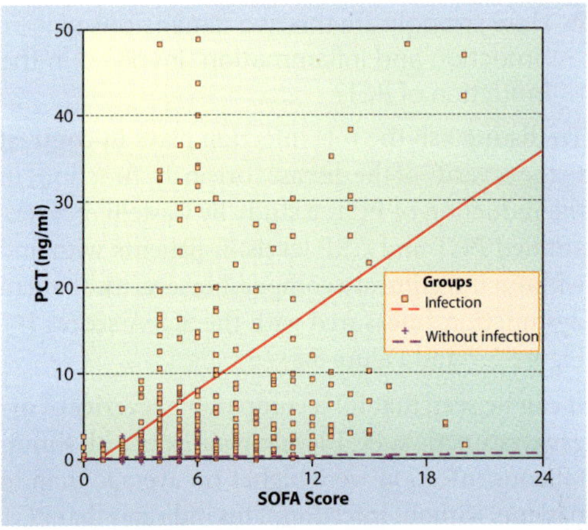

Figure 5.7: PCT concentration in patients in intensive care, with or without infections, as a function of the severity of organ dysfunction measured using the SOFA score. Graph of the regression lines for patients with infection (PCT = –0.84 + 1.526 × SOFA score, ng/ml) and without infection (PCT = 0.27 + 0.02 × SOFA score, ng/ml, p<0.02) (6).

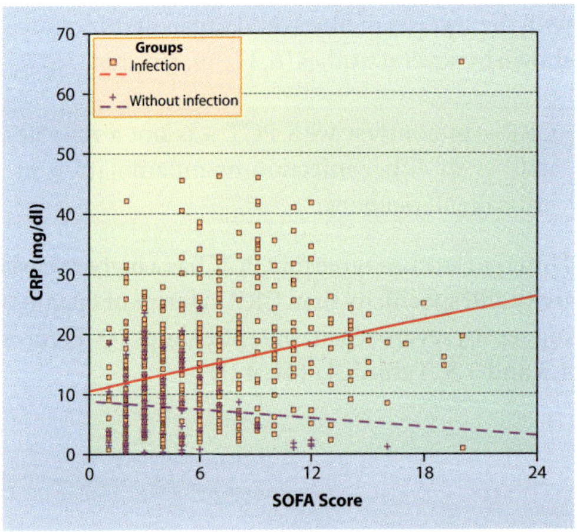

Figure 5.8: CRP concentration in patients in intensive care, with or without infections, as a function of the severity of organ dysfunction measured using the SOFA score. Graph of the regression lines for patients with infection (CRP = 105.58 + 0.72 × SOFA score. mg/l) and without infection (CRP = 84.53 – 0.19 × SOFA score. mg/l. p<0.001) (6).

5.5. Comparison with other markers

Most measurements of inflammation used in routine diagnosis are – in comparison with PCT – not specific to the diagnosis of sepsis. Besides the clinical signs and conventional measurement values (leukocyte counts, coagulation values, lactate), in particular CRP, IL-6, and to a certain extent LBP and the detection of bacterial endotoxins are used as markers of sepsis.

Important characteristics of these measurement values are listed below in comparison with PCT.

C-reactive protein (CRP)

CRP is an acute-phase protein synthesized in the liver during infections and different other inflammatory illnesses. An important stimulus for the formation of CRP is interleukin-6 (IL-6). CRP plays a role in the immune response, among other ways, as opsonin in the elimination of bacteria.

A serum level of more than 10 mg/l is generally expected for the diagnosis of an infection. Starting at concentrations of over 40 to 100 mg/l, a severe infection or sepsis can be anticipated. However, such concentrations can also occur in other illnesses, e.g. postoperative, or after a trauma. CRP values in patients with sepsis, severe sepsis, and septic shock often fall between 200 and 500 mg/l.

Significant differences between CRP and PCT:

- The kinetics of induction and elimination of CRP are significantly slower than for PCT or cytokines (order of magnitude of days instead of hours).
- CRP correlates only slightly with the severity of the sepsis. The marker thus cannot detect a progression to severe sepsis.
- As a result, the correlation with the progression of the illness, the prognosis (or risk), and the mortality of the illness in different situations (sepsis, trauma) is weak or nonexistent.
- CRP may be a sensitive marker for inflammatory stimuli, but it is relatively nonspecific: elevated levels can also be seen in different non-bacterially induced illnesses, e.g. viral infections, autoimmune diseases, local infections.
- The formation of CRP can be changed under immune suppression.

The designation of CRP as a "sepsis marker" or the measurement of CRP alone for the diagnosis of sepsis can therefore not be recommended in critically ill patients.

PCT			CRP			Number of patients	Literature
Cutoff (ng/ml)	Sensitivity (%)	Specificity (%)	Cutoff (mg/l)	Sensitivity (%)	Specificity (%)		
0.8	68	48	154	50	74	208	(121)
0.6	68	62	79	72	67	190	(105)
2	96	86	—	—	—	185	(134)
1.11	79	85	128	67	82	150	(6)
1	94	64	—	—	—	119	(135)
2	91	89	—	—	—	108	(136)
1	89	94	100	71	78	101	(13)
2	65	70	100	74	74	95	(119)
1.3	73	83	39	35	42	85	(15)
1.1	97	78	150	68	73	78	(33)
1	95	54	—	—	—	75	(17)

Table 5.4: Sensitivity and specificity of PCT and CRP in the diagnosis of sepsis, severe sepsis, or septic shock. Clinical studies with more than 75 patients were selected for the table. Studies are excluded that were performed on patients after a trauma or surgical intervention (according to (42)).

The differences in detail can be listed as follows:

- Delayed time behavior of induction and elimination of CRP

After a defined trauma, the maximum levels of CRP are only reached after 2 or 3 days, and normalization of the serum level takes several days, sometimes over a week, even though the biological half-life of the protein itself is only about a day (☞ Figure 3.4, Figure 5.10). These kinetics are insufficient for today's requirements for modern sepsis diagnosis.

- Lack of correlation of CRP with the severity of the illness

CRP values only have a slight relationship with the severity of the illness (☞ Figure 1.4, Table 5.4, Table 8.2) (6, 12, 105, 367). Many patients in intensive care, but also patients after operations or a trauma, have elevated CRP levels without the presence of severe sepsis. The correlation with the SOFA score is low (6, 367). Patients with severe illnesses cannot therefore be reliably distinguished from patients with only slight risk. A diagnosis of severe sepsis could be missed.

- Low specificity of CRP for a diagnosis of sepsis

CRP is not only induced in autoimmune diseases and viral infections. Elevated levels can be detected even after smaller surgical interventions or a trauma (☞ Section 8.2., Figure 8.2, Table 8.2). Values of over 100 mg/dl can easily occur. Concentrations correlate only slightly with the later progression and prognosis of the illness (21, 129, 130). They generally remain elevated for several days (☞ Figures 5.9 and 5.10). A reliable postoperative diagnosis of infection or sepsis is thus impossible with CRP, since infections often occur when CRP is already elevated postoperatively. On the other hand, given a complication-free progression, PCT already decreases after the first day post-op, if it is elevated at all (☞ Figure 5.9, Table 8.2) (21, 131, 132).

PCT is a marker which reacts more quickly than CRP, reflects severity, progression, and prognosis of the disease better than CRP, and is more specific for infection and sepsis than CRP.

Indications for measurement of CRP should therefore not depend on questions involving the specificity of the marker or the evaluation of the severity of sepsis. Since CRP reacts in some cases even to a relatively small systemic inflammatory response – unlike PCT – CRP is often used in outpatient care and as a general, non-specific indicator of inflammatory diseases. In the ultrasensitive range (concentrations under 1 to 4 mg/l), CRP is a risk indicator for coronary vascular events (133). In patients in intensive care, on the other hand, its informational content is limited.

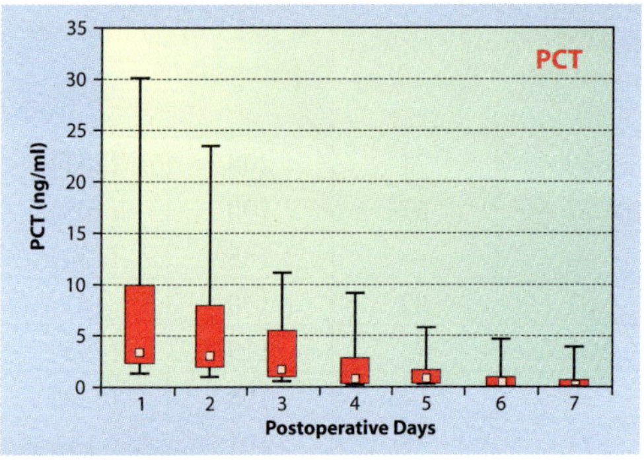

Figure 5.9: Time behavior of PCT values (ng/ml) in patients after heart surgery with complications (n=64). The median (dot), quartile (box), and 10/90 percentile (bar) are given (137).

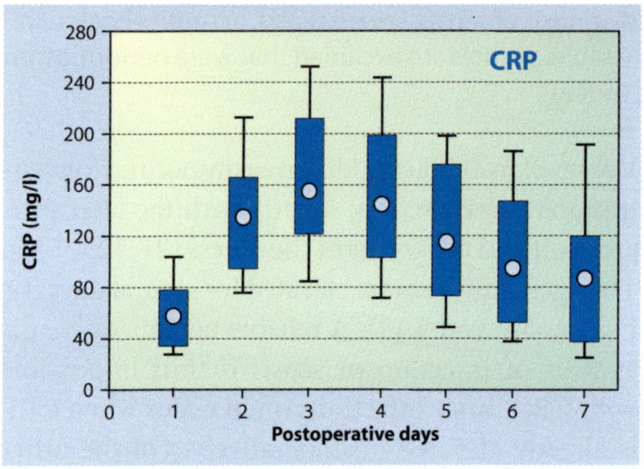

Figure 5.10: Time behavior of CRP values (ng/ml) in patients after heart surgery with complications (n=64). The median (dot), quartile (box), and 10/90 percentile (bar) are given (137).

Interleukin 6 (IL-6)

Interleukin 6 (IL-6) is a proinflammatory cytokine. Cytokines are proteins that act as messengers to carry information about inflammations to other cells. IL-6 is synthesized by different types of cells, particularly monocytary cells of the blood (acute stimulation) and endothelial cells (for illness of longer duration).

Measurable concentrations range from a few pg/ml (normal range) to levels of over 1000 pg/ml for severe sepsis or multiple organ failure. Induction takes place quickly after stimulation of these cells (within one to a few hours). IL-6 is also measurable in the case of local infections – in contrast to PCT – in bruises and other tissue fluids (BAL, pleural contusion, joint contusions). In contrast with PCT, no other cell-to-cell interactions are necessary for induction. Endotoxins and different cytokines directly cause IL-6 production – even in a blood sample already taken – and both bacterial and viral infections or autoimmune processes and tissue trauma trigger induction. IL-6 is thus not an infection-specific marker.

Elevated IL-6 levels decrease correspondingly quickly. Thus greatly variable plasma levels can occur, the interpretation of which is often not simple. It must also be considered that the synthesis of IL-6 and other cytokines is partly suppressed by immune suppression. In patients subject to immune suppression IL-6 levels must therefore be interpreted with care.

When drawing and transporting blood, a few specific things must be noted: full blood drawn must be cooled and centrifuged quickly, and the containers used must be free of endotoxins, since otherwise IL-6 can decompose or be formed by leukocytes in the blood sample.

Although there are currently no suitable meta-analyses and individual studies indicate a less clear correlation (138), it can be assumed that the plasma level of IL-6 in sepsis or after operative trauma correlates relatively well with severity, and to a certain extent also with the prognosis for the illness (138). Persistently elevated plasma levels of over 1000 pg/ml are often considered an indication of an unfavorable progression or mortality outcome (139).

In pediatrics, IL-6 has become favored as a sepsis marker, since IL-6 reacts very quickly and high levels occur quickly in newborns and small children. A more detailed analysis of the existing studies, however, shows that PCT is also highly sensitive and specific for the diagnosis of sepsis on first contact with the physician or admission to the hospital even in newborns and small children, and that it is not inferior to other markers. The time factor is thus no disadvantage to PCT even in these patients (☞ Chapter 9.3., Table 9.1).

Endotoxin

Endotoxin has been discussed for a long time as a possible marker of sepsis. Sufficiently sensitive detection of endotoxin in infections and sepsis, however, has become possible only recently. The "endotoxin activity assay" permits the detection of endotoxinemia in an "ultrasensitive" range (140). However, the test is difficult, since fresh full blood must be examined in a kinetic measurement series. The value also correlates only slightly with the clinical severity of the sepsis (140). Additional studies are still needed to demonstrate the clinical usefulness of this test.

Other markers

Different markers for infection and inflammation have been presented in the past few years. These include sTREM-1 (soluble triggering receptor expressed on myeloid cells), MBL (mannan-binding lectin), copeptin, Macrophage Migration Inhibitory Factor (MIF), Lipopolysaccharide-Binding Protein (LBP), leukocyte surface markers such as HLA-DR, and the endotoxin activity assay (141-146).

Many of these markers exhibit a high diagnostic sensitivity or specificity in terms of diagnosis of an infection in cases of limited questions or in special patient populations. Clinical reference to the severity of the illness, however, which in the end enables an evaluation of the progression, is lacking in the markers listed. This is also true of markers in the coagulation system, which can also be used as sensitive diagnostic and prognostic markers of sepsis (147).

New measurements which correlate better with the severity or risk of illness, however, are less specific for bacterial infections. These measurements include, for example, MR-proadrenomedullin (MR-proADM), copeptin, and for certain questions, MR-proANP (148, 149). If a combination of markers of bacterial infection and risk-associated markers or indicators of cardiac insufficiency is used, unclear diagnostic situations can often be better differentiated than with the exclusive use of conventional diagnostics (359).

Many new markers of infection and inflammation must still be proven in clinical practice, or must be subjected to additional clinical trials. Only a few address the aspects important for routine use in clinical practice. These requirements include a clear indication and detectable diagnostic advantage for the treating physician, but also basic characteristics such as high stability in the blood sample, a clinically acceptable half-life, and simple measurement methods. Only when these factors coincide is a new laboratory chemical measurement clinically useful.

6. Use of PCT for the control of antibiotic therapy

6.1. Basics of an individual, patient-adapted antibiotic treatment using PCT

▶ Goals of an individual, patient-adapted antibiotic therapy ("IPAT")

The goal of a modern anti-infective therapy is the adaptation of treatment to the individual requirements of the patient. This includes a well-founded indication, an individually-adapted duration of treatment, and changes to the antibiotic in case of insufficient effectiveness. Only daily monitoring of the indications can prevent unnecessary treatment and thus an increased rate of development of resistance and side effects. Basic requirements and goals for an individual, patient-adapted antibiotic treatment are shown in Tables 6.1 and 2.2.

Immunological markers like PCT open up new paths to patient-oriented, risk-adapted treatment, since they offer an increased reliability profile (infection diagnosis, sepsis diagnosis, evaluation of the risk profile for organ dysfunction and mortality). Different studies have shown that PCT – in combination with clinical data – can improve the indications for antibiotic treatment and optimize the necessary duration of treatment. Thus PCT level measurement increases diagnostic reliability for detecting and specifically treating patients with severe bacterial infections or sepsis requiring treatment. Moreover, when using a PCT-controlled treatment algorithm, the duration of antibiotic treatment can be reduced by an average of at least two days – even for patients with sepsis or severe sepsis. An analysis of the studies available shows that starting from a duration of treatment of 5 to 7 days, a possible termination of antibiotic treatment, depending on the success of therapy, should be considered (☞ Figures 6.6 and 6.9) (23, 25, 356, 369).

Statistical records show that antibiotic usage differs greatly, not just between countries, but also within individual countries, e.g. between different intensive care units. This data indicates that the practical rules for use of antibiotics differ from place to place (☞ Figures 6.1 and 6.2) (46, 47, 150). Since antibiotic use is unambiguously related to the development of resistant bacterial strains and the frequency of occurrence of undesirable side effects, there is a need for action in checking the criteria used to prescribe antibiotics, not only scientifically but also in everyday use (45, 46).

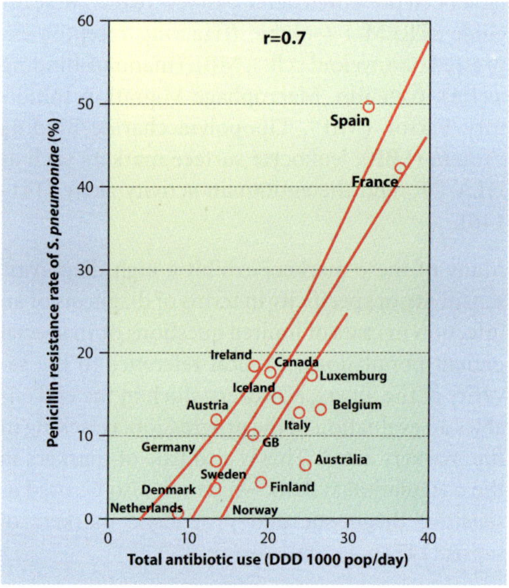

Figure 6.1: Example of a correlation between the average rate of prescription of antibiotics and the number of resistant isolates. The relationship between the resistance rate of *Streptococcus pneumoniae* to penicillin and the average use of antibiotics in Europe (46).

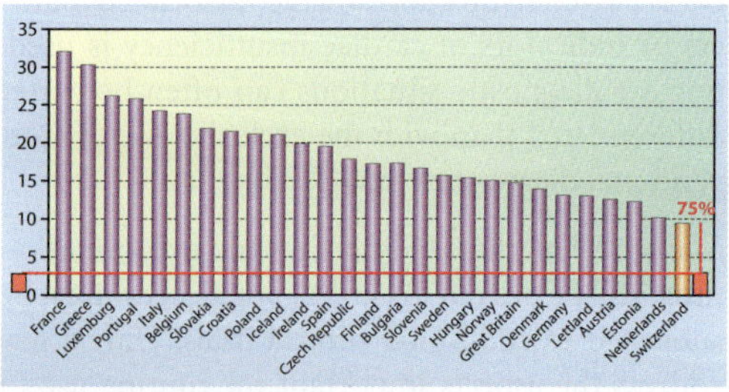

Figure 6.2: Frequency of prescription of antibiotics in different countries (average daily dosages per 1000 inhabitants). Despite the relatively low usage, a reduction in the rate of prescription of more than 70% was possible due to PCT-controlled therapy in one study in Switzerland (47).

When prescribing antibiotics, we should first be clear on the basis of what indication and due to which infection the medicine is prescribed. This decision should be documented in the patient's file – if possible on a separate sheet ("antibiotic progression sheet"). There are different reasons for the prescription of antibiotics (☞ Section 2.1.5. and Table 2.2). Many of these fall into the area of "convenience" – or of increased notions of safety in case of unclear or unconfirmed diagnoses (☞ Table 2.2). This also applies to so-called "prophylactic treatment". In outpatient care, the actual diagnosis of "sepsis" is only rarely cause for treatment. Only a few treatments are truly necessary to prevent locally destructive effects or lingering damage to individual organs. Patients not eligible for an individually patient-adapted and PCT-controlled therapy progression monitoring must be identified. These include, for example, infections with locally destructive effects or a lack of self-limitation of the illness (endocarditis, local cerebral infections or abscess, osteomyelitis), infections with certain agents (e.g. tuberculosis), or patients with weakened immune systems (hematological oncology, chemotherapy, immune suppression, severe inflammatory illnesses, etc.) (☞ Section 2.1.5., Tables 2.2 and 6.1).

Different studies have shown that an individual, patient-adapted, PCT-controlled antibiotic therapy in stationary patients permits a reduction in the duration of treatment of at least 2 days, and for outpatient care, a reduction in the frequency of treatment by at least some 50% is possible.

Individual, Patient-adapted, Antibiotic Treatment (IPAT)
• Is based on the basic idea of treating only specific periods of severe infections requiring treatment. - And this only as long as clinically necessary. - The identification of a specific bacterially inflammatory focus must be attempted and documented. - The reason for administration of antibiotics, including the case history of antibiotics, must be documented.
• Requires the measurement of markers of inflammation and infection in order to achieve increased diagnostic reliability (e.g. diagnosis of sepsis).
• Requires an intensified sepsis monitoring in patients receiving no antibiotics.
• The clinical success of the treatment has top priority, while the treatment of microbial findings should be considered, but has lower priority.
• De-escalation strategies are generally unnecessary, since the duration of treatment is always held as low as possible and is limited to the success of therapy.
• The ability of the organism to fight infection ("immune competence") must always be present. - The treatment of immune-compromised patients or patients with severe SIRS, MODS, or elevated PCT levels due to non-bacterial causes with IPAT is not recommended, or should be done only with increased care. - High PCT levels – even with no evidence of infection – are an indication of a problem with the specific immune function of the patient (e.g. a problem with the intestinal barrier function, bacterial translocation, microperfusion problems) and should also be considered an indication needed antibacterial treatment even in patients with no evidence of infection.
• There are indications that IPAT reduces the cost of antibiotic therapy without significantly changing mortality. This, and the question of whether fewer resistances emerge under IPAT, must be examined in additional studies, however.

Table 6.1: The goals and requirements of an individual, patient-adapted antibiotic treatment (IPAT).

The goal of a modern anti-infective therapy is the adaptation of treatment to the individual requirements of the patient (indications, duration of treatment, if necessary a change in antibiotics).
Immunological markers such as PCT open up new diagnostic paths to a patient-oriented, risk-adapted treatment, since they can detect severe bacterial infection or sepsis in a patient with high diagnostic reliability.

▶ What studies are there of PCT-controlled antibiotic therapy?

Numerous studies in the past few years have addressed the questions of a PCT-controlled antibiotic treatment (☞ Table 6.2). These include both outpatient care and patients in intensive care, for example patients with airway infections (22, 44), COPD (24), community-acquired pneumonia (23), or general patients in intensive care with a diagnosis of sepsis or severe sepsis (25, 356, 369). In these studies, a reduction in the duration of treatment or in the rate of prescription was observed, usually on the order of at least 2 days of therapy (25, 23, 34, 108, 151-154, 356, 359). An overview of the indications and treatment algorithms of corresponding studies can be found in Table 6.2. PCT level measurement and the use of corresponding treatment algorithms to monitor the necessity of antibiotic treatment have also proved useful in daily clinical practice. However, it is still recommended observing certain basic requirements when controlling antibiotic therapy with PCT.

▶ Basic rules for the interpretation of PCT for an individual, patient-adapted antibiotic therapy

▶ **1.** An individual, PCT-controlled treatment must be indicated.

Locally destructive processes, processes with a lack of self-limitation, illnesses with special agents or a potential hazard to the patient must be excluded (e.g. endocarditis, meningitis, meningococcal infections, tuberculosis) (☞ Tables 2.2 and 6.1). Patients with a weakened immune defense should be treated with particular care.

▶ **2.** The clinical findings must be noted.

In any case, clinical, radiological, and laboratory chemical signs must be used in addition to PCT to evaluate the effectiveness or necessity of antibiotic treatment.

These include, for example:

- Local findings (local signs of infection, X-ray findings, e.g. decrease in infiltrates, changes in secretion)
- Progression of other signs of systemic inflammatory response (e.g. fever, leukocyte counts)
- Signs of organ dysfunction (catecholoamine requirement, progression of oxygenation, coagulation values).

▶ **3.** The clinical symptoms of suspected or proven infection should be registered.

Generally, laboratory measurements should be taken only if a specific question is posed. Hence, the clinical diagnosis and purpose of PCT measurement and antibiotic therapy should be known and registered (e.g. treatment of pneumonia, source control after focus removal in patients with peritonitis or leakage of anastomosis). Possible questions for PCT in the context of control of an antibiotic regimen might be:

At the onset of an illness:

- Is there a focus of the infection?
- Is there local infection only or already symptoms of systemic inflammation?
- Is antibiotic treatment necessary or not?
- What is the reason for treatment?

During therapy:

- Is the antibiotic treatment effective or not and must the antibiotic be replaced with another?
- When can an antibiotic treatment be discontinued or is the patient still in danger of a systemic inflammatory response?

▶ **4.** General aspects of PCT trends must be observed.

Falling PCT levels approaching the normal range are generally signs of a good prognosis. Increasing or persistently elevated PCT values are often signs of a poor prognosis (12, 20, 36, 38, 155-157). Moreover, the absolute value of the PCT level can provide indications of a possible danger to the patient from sepsis or due to a severe bacterial infection. Possible non-specific causes of PCT induction should be known and taken into consideration (e.g. severe chronic kidney insufficiency, severe liver insufficiency, postoperative induction) (☞ Sections 8.1. and 8.4.).

In detail, this means:

- It is unlikely for very low PCT levels to be associated with the presence of severe bacterial infections or sepsis. The high negative predictive value of low PCT levels (particularly when PCT <0.1 ng/ml) can therefore be used to exclude a severe bacterial infection or sepsis – if this data can be reconciled with the clinical findings. Local infections may occur, but are generally not threatening. The probability of isolating positive blood cultures is rather low for normal PCT levels.
- Elevated PCT levels indicate a diagnosis of sepsis with increasing probability. The high positive predictive value of highly elevated PCT levels for this diagnosis can be interpreted as an indication of the urgent necessity of antibiotic treatment or focal surgery. Here, too, the probability of isolating positive blood cultures is higher for high PCT levels.
- When interpreting PCT levels, refer to the corresponding general and special sections as well as to the explanation for FDA approval in the United States (☞ Sections 1.4., 2.1.1. and 2.1.4.).

> The trend of PCT levels can give an indication of the progression of the disease and the effectiveness of therapy.
> The absolute value of the current PCT level is significant in this process.

If the clinical findings remain unclear or if they cannot reliably exclude a severe bacterial infection, the following basic rules apply:

- A PCT level of less than 0.1 ng/ml (depending on clinical circumstances, even one less than 0.25 ng/ml) is a factor against beginning antibiotic treatment.
- A PCT level of over 0.5 ng/ml indicates possible sepsis or severe bacterial infection, and is thus a factor in favor of antibiotic treatment as long as no other diagnosis explains the elevated levels. In outpatients also PCT levels >0.25 ng/ml may indicate infection.

When evaluating the effectiveness of antibiotic treatment, then in addition to clinical data, PCT levels provide indications of the effectiveness of treatment:

- If PCT levels fall within the first 72 hours (generally a reduction by more than 30% in comparison with the previous day's level) then the treatment is generally effective. The antibiotics selected should in that case be continued (taking the current resistogram into consideration).
- If PCT levels do not fall within the first few days of treatment, this indicates some doubt as to the effectiveness of the therapy. A possible change in or extension of the antibiotic treatment should be discussed, and reconciled with the clinical findings.

With respect to the duration of antibiotic treatment:

- The duration of antibiotic treatment is always based on the currently valid guidelines. However, it must be noted that every treatment lasting longer than 7 days must be considered questionable in terms of its effectiveness. A longer duration of treatment should therefore be the exception. In some illnesses or after successful elimination of the focus of infection (pneumonia, urinary tract infection, removal of an infected catheter), even after a shorter duration of treatment (e.g. after the third but no later than the fifth day of treatment) it should be asked whether antibiotic treatment is still required (151, 152). Thus, if the PCT levels fall by more than 90% from the baseline, consideration may be given to stopping the antibiotic therapy (23).
- It is decisive for the interpretation of PCT that a persistent, clear reduction of PCT must be observed, that the focus of the illness be healed, and that systemic inflammatory response be clearly reduced or eliminated (☞ point 2).
- Longer treatment periods require a rational, individual reason (e.g. bacterial endocarditis, osteomyelitis, tuberculosis, difficult-to-access abscessing infections; ☞ also Table 2.2 and (25)).
- In case of doubt, the situation must be reevaluated, e.g. detection of agent, antibiotic-free period, change in antibiotic treatment, change in strategy of focal elimination.

<table>
<tr><th>Illness, inclusion criteria</th><th>Treatment algorithm</th><th>Result</th><th>Literature, no. of pat.</th></tr>
<tr><td colspan="4">Outpatients and intensive care patients</td></tr>
<tr><td rowspan="2">Patients with cough, dyspnea in the emergency clinic with suspicion of infection of lower airways</td><td rowspan="4">**PCT <0.1 ng/ml:** A severe bacterial infection requiring therapy is improbable: prescription of antibiotics not at all recommended
PCT 0.1-0.25 ng/ml: A bacterial infection requiring therapy is not probable: antibiotic therapy not recommended
PCT 0.25-0.5 ng/ml: A bacterial infection requiring therapy may be present: antibiotic therapy recommended
PCT >0.5 ng/ml: An infection requiring therapy is probable: antibiotic therapy is strongly recommended.
For patients already taking antibiotics upon admission: if PCT <0.25 ng/ml: discontinuation of the antibiotics recommended.
Also in (385) (ProHOSP): discontinuation of antibiotic therapy recommended if more than an 80% decrease compared with baseline value (90%, strongly recommended)</td><td>Reduction in rate of prescription per 1000 days of observation: 661/1000 vs. 332/1000 (83% vs. 44%).</td><td>(22), n=243</td></tr>
<tr><td>A shorter duration of treatment with antibiotics in the PCT-guided group (5.7 vs. 8.7 days) with the same outcome but fewer side effects</td><td>(385) n=1359</td></tr>
<tr><td>Antibiotic treatment considered by general practitioner in patients with suspicion of acute airway infections of various types</td><td>Reduction in frequency of prescription by more than 70%</td><td>(44), n=458</td></tr>
<tr><td>Acute exacerbation of a COPD</td><td>Reduction in rate of prescription: 40% vs. 72% (study/control group)</td><td>(24), n=208</td></tr>
<tr><td colspan="4">Inpatient treatment and patients in intensive care</td></tr>
<tr><td>Community-acquired pneumonia (CAP), any severity</td><td>Criteria as above.</td><td>Shorter duration of treatment in the PCT group: 5 days vs. 12 days (median of study/control group)</td><td>(23), n=302</td></tr>
<tr><td>Severe sepsis, septic shock</td><td>For a "base value" (peak value) of ≥1 ng/ml: follow-up on day 5. End of antibiosis if PCT <10% of the base value or absolute value <0.25 ng/ml.
For base value <1 ng/ml: check on day 3: end of antibiosis of PCT <0.1 ng/ml. If blood culture positive: Treatment at least 5 days.</td><td>Reduction in duration of antibiotic treatment: 6 days vs. 9.5 days (median of study/control group)</td><td>(25), n=79</td></tr>
<tr><td>Patients in operative intensive care with sepsis (at least 2 SIRS criteria = severe sepsis, septic shock)</td><td>Discontinuation of antibiotic therapy after reduction in clinical signs of infection and PCT ≤1 ng/ml or (if PCT >1 ng/ml) if reduction after 3 days to 25-35% of the starting level (=decrease of more than 65-75% in 3 days)</td><td>Shorter duration of antibiotic treatment (2 days) in the PCT group (5.9 ± 1.7 vs. 7.9 ± 0.5 days)
Shorter duration of intensive treatment in the PCT group</td><td>(356), n=110</td></tr>
<tr><td>Patients with severe sepsis</td><td>Discontinuation of antibiotic therapy if regression of clinical signs of infection and PCT ≤1 ng/ml or (if PCT >1 ng/ml) if decrease after 3 days to 25-35% of the baseline value.</td><td>Shorter duration of treatment by 1.7 days in the PCT group (6.6 ± 1.1 vs. 8.3 ± 0.7 days)</td><td>(369), n=27</td></tr>
</table>

Inpatient treatment and patients in intensive care (continued)			
Patients in intensive care with suspected infections, multicentre study	**PCT <0.25 ng/ml or >0.25 to <0.5 ng/ml:** antibiotic therapy not recommended (stronger or less strong recommendation, respectively) **PCT >0.5 to <1 ng/ml or >1 ng/ml:** Antibiotic therapy recommended (clear or compelling need, respectively) **Course:** if PCT falls to below 80 % of the peak value or falls to <0.5 ng/ml: Discontinuation of antibiotic therapy recommended based on the PCT values.	Antibiotic-free days (observation period 28 days, study primary end point): PCT: 14.3±9.0 days, control: 11.6±8.2 days (23% relative reduction in antibiotic exposure), no difference in mortality	(389), n=621
Ventilator-associated pneumonia (VAP), 5 centers	**PCT after 72 hours:** <0.25 ng/ml or PCT >0.25 ng/ml to <0.5 ng/ml or more than 80% decrease compared with day 0: discontinuation of antibiotic therapy is recommended (strong or less strong recommendation, respectively). **PCT ≥0.5 ng/ml or less than 80% decrease or PCT >1 ng/ml:** discontinuation of antibiotic therapy is not recommended (level of recommendation, less strong or strong, respectively). Daily re-evaluation after 72 hours.	Antibiotic-free days (28-day observation period): 13 days (PCT) vs 9.5 days (control group), 27% relative reduction in antibiotic treatment (study primary end point). Secondary end points (risk assessment): no differences between the groups (mortality, treatment days with ventilation or in intensive care)	(371), n=101

Table 6.2: Overview of studies controlling antibiotic therapy using PCT. The rate of complications was identical between the study and control groups in all studies.

- A de-escalation strategy is usually unnecessary in this system, since the treatment period is already as short as possible.

6.2. PCT-controlled antibiotic therapy in airway infections

6.2.1. Overview of current studies

Studies of PCT-controlled antibiotic therapy with an interventional strategy were first carried out in patients with infections of the airway (symptoms "dyspnea and coughing" in the emergency room). Later on studies considering patients with COPD and pneumonia followed (23, 24). The workgroup of Prof. Beat Müller in Switzerland were pioneers in this area. In the meantime, other research groups have joined the plan, and carried out PCT-controlled interventional studies on patients in intensive care and on newborns (☞ Table 6.1). Airway infections are particularly suitable for PCT-controlled monitoring, since the spectrum of possible illnesses is very broad and since the mortality rate for simple infections is low. The spectrum of illnesses ranges from mild bacterial or non-bacterially caused illnesses, in which no antibiotic treatment is indicated (bronchitis, laryngitis, tracheitis, pharyngitis, often due to viral agents, sometimes with superinfections), to patients with chronic obstructive pulmonary disease (COPD) and patients with pneumonia of various degrees of severity and with different causes. Here, with the exception of demonstrated pneumonia, the treating physician is often not certain whether an antibiotic should be prescribed or not, and how long the optimum duration of treatment would be (151-154, 158).

The basis for most of the treatment algorithms used in these studies is the observation that for "normal" PCT levels (PCT below 0.1 ng/ml) there is only a very low risk of severe infection or sepsis, while for PCT levels above 0.5 ng/ml the risk to the patient of sepsis or severe bacterial infection cannot be excluded (☞ Table 6.1 and Figure 6.3).

In the studies listed, therefore, a very low threshold for PCT was generally used to exclude infection (0.1 ng/ml to 0.25 ng/ml). Only in this way can high sensitivity and the high negative predictive value of PCT can be used to exclude septic complications. Since not all PCT assays provide sufficient accuracy in this measurement range, the func-

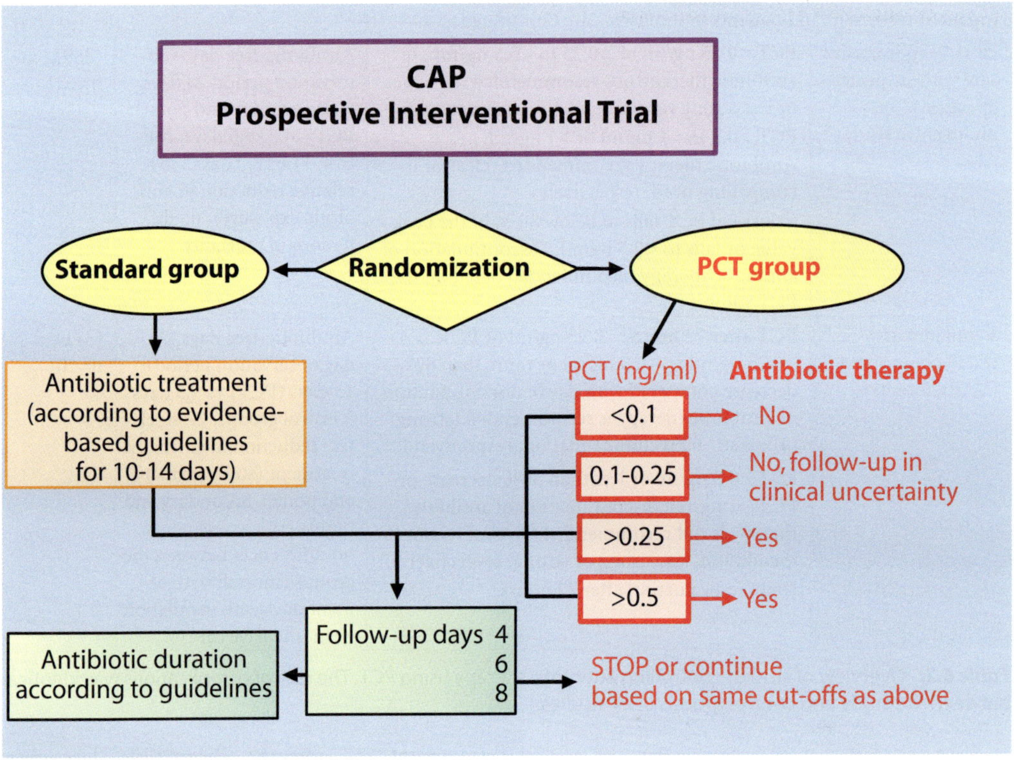

Figure 6.3: Decision algorithm for an individual, patient-adapted antibiotic therapy in patients with community-acquired pneumonia in a prospective, randomized study. Very low PCT levels are – in combination with clinical data – an indication to discontinue antibiotic therapy (23).

tional assay sensitivity of the measurement method used should be checked before use. It should be under 0.1 ng/ml (☞ also Section 4.1.).

For intensive care patients, on the other hand, different but essentially very similar algorithms were used. Here, the relative decrease in relation to the baseline value was included in the assessment, so that antibiotic treatment of certain patients – if focal elimination seems likely from a clinical standpoint as well – can be discontinued even for higher limit values.

In the studies listed, PCT was able to reduce the rate of prescription and duration of treatment with antibiotics significantly, without complications occurring more frequently (22).

Selected studies are presented below.

6.2.2. Patients with suspicion of infections of the upper airways in the emergency room: the "ProResp" study

This study included 243 patients who attended the emergency room with the symptoms "dyspnea and cough" and who were deemed by the physician to be candidates for antibiotic therapy after detailed clinical examination ("ProResp" study, ☞ Table 6.1and 6.2) (22). The control group was treated conventionally without PCT measurement (119 patients). In the study group, the physician acted in the knowledge of PCT levels and a PCT-controlled recommendation for or against the prescription of antibiotics. The rate of prescription of antibiotics in the PCT group was 44%, versus 83% in the control group (☞ Figure 6.4).

The greatest reduction in antibiotic use was observed in patients with illnesses not always requiring antibiotic treatment (e.g. bronchitis or asthma). Patients with pneumonia, on the other hand – as expected – received antibiotics in nearly all cases (☞ Figure 6.4). Diagnostic reliability was thus increased by PCT measurement (22).

This reduction in antibiotic use caused no observable increase in the rate of complications. It also resulted in a reduction in costs.

> In patients with airway infections and the symptoms "coughing and dyspnea", the use of a PCT-controlled treatment algorithm was able to reduce the rate of prescription of antibiotics by almost half.

	Standard group	PCT group
Received antibiotic	83%	44%
Duration of antibiotic therapy	12.8 days	10.9 days
Number of days of stationary treatment	11.2 days	10.7 days
Intensive treatment needed	5%	4%
Deaths	3%	3%
Antibiotic costs per patient	USD $202	USD $96

Table 6.3: The results of the "ProResp" study (22). Data is listed on the frequency and duration of antibiotic treatment, as well as the duration of hospital stay for patients with suspicion of airway infections treated according to conventional points of view (standard group) and patients treated according to a PCT-controlled treatment algorithm (☞ Table 6.1) (22).

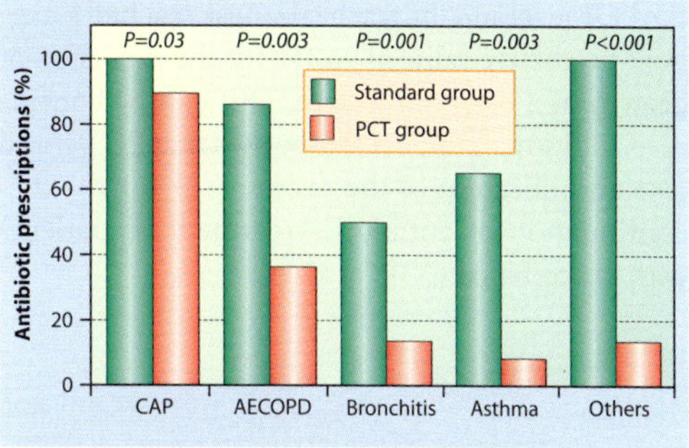

Figure 6.4: Reduction in the rate of prescription of antibiotics – categorized retrospectively into different diagnoses – in patients treated in the emergency room for symptoms of "coughing and dyspnea" with a suspicion of infections in the lower airways, comparing a control group (no PCT measurement) with the PCT group (PCT level measurement and use of a recommendation algorithm for antibiotic treatment, a so-called "ProResp" study) (22).

6.2.3. PCT, antibiotic therapy, and exacerbation of COPD: the "ProCOLD" study

Antibiotics are often prescribed for exacerbation of chronic bronchitis, as well, without the usefulness of this treatment being unambiguously clear. When using a PCT-controlled treatment algorithm, the frequency of prescription of antibiotics in the acute phase of the illness was only 40%, while without PCT measurement it was 72% (control group) (24). The effect observed was also significant over a 6-month observation period, without complications arising more frequently (no higher mortality, hospitalization, or reinfection rate) (☞ Figure 6.5). The use of a highly sensitive measurement procedure is important here, as well (analytical assay sensitivity about 0.1 ng/ml), since PCT generally reacts to simple bacterial infections only with a slight increase which is barely above the normal range. In one study from China, under a limit value of just 0.15 ng/ml, the sensitivity of detection of an infection was more than 93%. The specificity for diagnosis at that value was 60% (159). Additional studies on patients with severe exacerbation of COPD have shown that PCT levels of more than 0.5 ng/ml or the presence of Gram-positive preparations in the tracheal aspirate were also associated with a positive bacterial culture in the aspirate (376). The sensitivity and specificity of this finding are low, but the combination of information about the PCT level and the tracheal smear reached a negative predictive value of 96.7% for the exclusion of growth of a bacterial isolate. This can be considered additional support for the idea that PCT could give an indication of the necessity or for the discontinuation of antibiotic treatment in patients with exacerbated COPD (376).

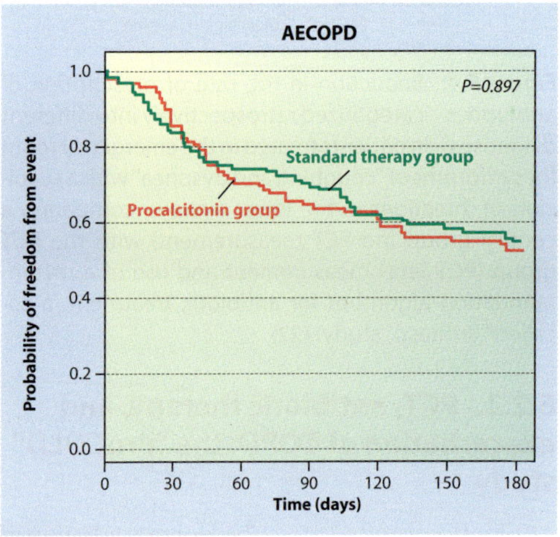

Figure 6.5: Kaplan-Meier curve of the probability of a relapse or survival 6 months after randomized treatment of patients with acute exacerbated chronic obstructive pulmonary disease (AECOPD).
Red line: procalcitonin group: only 40% of patients received antibiotics after admission, Green line: control group: 72% of patients in the control group received antibiotics for AECOPD upon admission (24).

6.2.4. Outpatients with suspicion of airway infections: the "PARTI" study

Many antibiotics are prescribed for outpatients for reasons of convenience or at the patient's request. These prescriptions are often grouped into a "convenience" category. For example, this includes prescriptions given for "symptom reduction" or "to shorten the duration of illness" (☞ Table 2.2). In these cases, there is no vital indication of risk of sepsis or danger of organ damage from locally destructive processes. The majority of bacterial infections treated on an outpatient basis (particularly infections of the airways) resolve without lasting damage even without antibiotic therapy. These include, for example, bronchitis, laryngotracheitis, otitis media, sometimes tonsillitis (if no streptococcus is detected) and – in some cases – even infections of soft tissue or uncomplicated urinary tract infections.

In a multicenter study in Switzerland, 8162 patients who visited physicians' offices with the suspicion of infection in acute airway infections were evaluated (44). In 458 patients, the physicians considered it necessary to prescribe an antibiotic based on the clinical symptoms. These patients were randomized. In the study group, the PCT value was measured and the physician was given a recommendation for or against antibiotic treatment based on an evaluation algorithm. For PCT values of less than 0.1 ng/ml or up to 0.25 ng/ml, this recommendation was against prescription; for levels of over 0.25 up to 0.5 ng/ml PCT was confirmed as the therapy recommendation. It was shown that in 72% of these patients, antibiotic treatment was not carried out after knowledge of the PCT level. It was also obviously unnecessary: the rate of complications was no higher in the PCT group. On the contrary: antibiotic-associated side effects such as diarrhea occurred significantly less frequently in the PCT group (44).

Thus by measuring PCT, the physician gains a tool to formulate the treatment and healing of the patient on a more goal-oriented basis. If there is suspicion of sepsis or severe infection, the necessity of antibiotic treatment can be clearly explained to the patient. If the treatment is unnecessary, a negative PCT value can help reduce the fear of complication from sepsis or severe bacterial infections, and explain to the patient the lack of urgency of treatment with antibiotics in comparison with the possible risks of antibiotic treatment (e.g. diarrhea, allergy). PCT level measurement thus represents an introduction to modern, rational, patient-oriented antibiotic treatment.

6.2.5. Individual, patient-adapted treatment of community-acquired pneumonia with PCT: the "ProCAP" study

In the antibiotic treatment of pneumonia, too, it makes sense to adapt the duration of treatment individually to the needs of the patient. For example, in community-acquired pneumonia (CAP) with low degree of severity or milder risk profile, a relatively short duration of treatment is possible (151). Here, too, PCT can support the clinical decision making process.

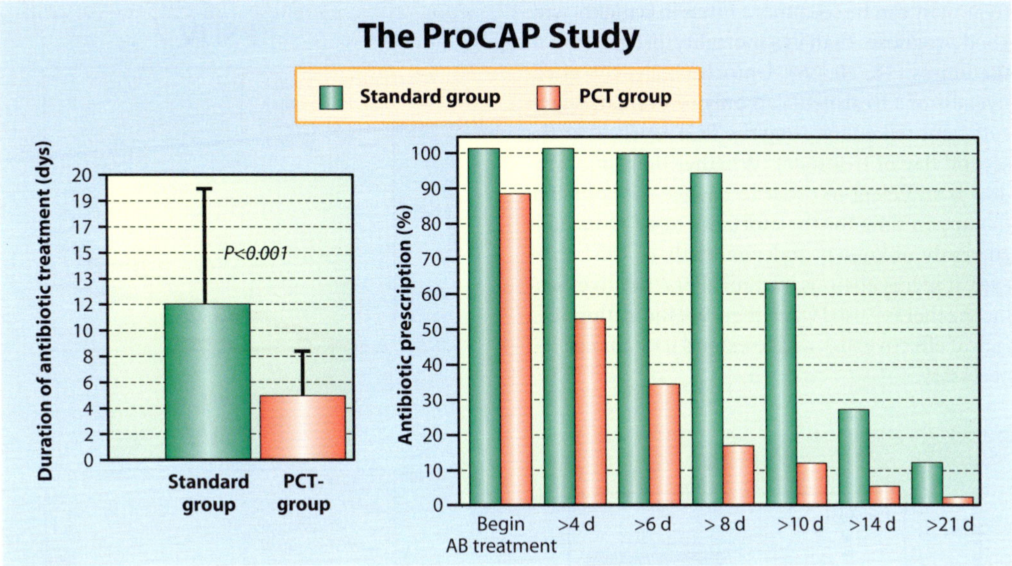

Figure 6.6: Duration of antibiotic therapy in patients with community-acquired pneumonia in the control group (green columns) and study group (red columns, PCT-supported treatment recommendations). The graph shows the percentage of patients treated with antibiotic on each day of treatment, as well as the average duration of treatment in the PCT and control groups (23).

Under study conditions, 302 patients with CAP were treated either conventionally or using a PCT-controlled treatment algorithm (☞ Table 6.1, Figure 6.3) (23). The duration of antibiotic treatment in the PCT-controlled group, with 5 days of treatment as compared to 12, was significantly shorter than with the conventional procedure (☞ Figures 6.6 and 6.7).

As expected, the largest reduction in the duration of treatment was in patients with low mortality risk of pneumonia ("Pneumonia Severity Index" (PSI) <III) and with negative blood cultures, while for severe pneumonia with an unfavorable risk profile (PSI classes IV and V) or in patients with a positive blood culture, the duration of treatment was also longer in the PCT group. The duration of treatment still seldom exceeded 7 to 8 days (exception: for bacteremia) (☞ Figure 6.7).

Other studies show that very low PCT levels in patients with pneumonia are an indication of a low mortality risk – sometimes unnoticed due to a high clinical risk profile (PSI III or IV) (☞ Figure 6.8) (35). Obviously, PCT also provides information describing the patient's risk profile.

The decision to discontinue an antibiotic treatment earlier or later can also be simplified by PCT level measurement.

> PCT levels – in addition to clinical criteria – can be used to adapt the duration of antibiotic therapy in community-acquired pneumonia better to the individual needs of the patient.

▶ Nosocomial pneumonias

In nosocomial pneumonia, it also seems possible to adapt the duration of treatment individually to the requirements of the patient, and thus generally to shorten them (152, 154, 158, 371). There is data indicating that – independently of PCT – the goal of a maximum duration of treatment of 7 to 8 days, depending on clinical findings, is a realistic goal (158, 371). Treatment cycles lasting less than 7 days are also possible, however.

> Besides the absolute level of PCT, in PCT-controlled antibiotic therapy the progression of PCT levels also plays an important role.

In different infection illnesses, including ventilator-associated pneumonia (VAP), it was observed that quickly declining PCT levels in the first days of treatment can be seen more often in patients with good prognoses than in a mortality progression of the illness (18, 20, 36). Unfortunately, the effectiveness of a treatment can only be evaluated with sufficient reliability using the PCT levels after the second day of treatment. Whether that time window is sufficient in order to change the course of therapy in time for the mortality to be reduced is currently unknown. Independently of this, however, it seems obvious in clinical practice to examine the therapy used when there are indications of a lack of effectiveness, and to extend it or change it if necessary.

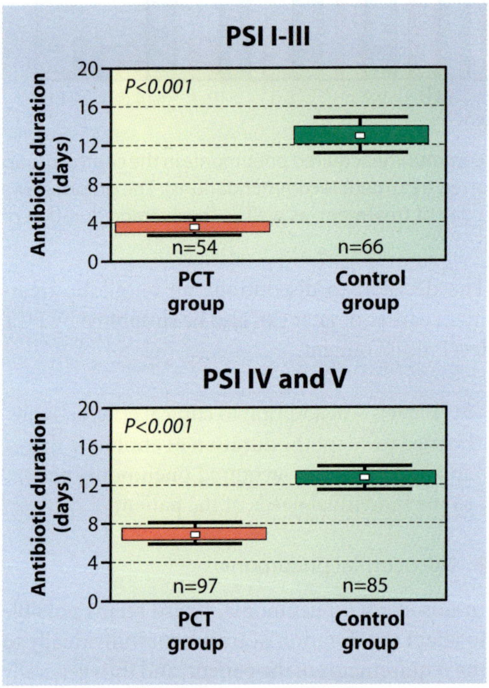

Figure 6.7: Duration of antibiotic therapy in patients with community-acquired pneumonia with a low risk profile (PSI I-III) and high risk profile (PSI IV+V). The graph shows the median levels and SEM (box) of the days of antibiotic treatment in patients treated according to fixed guidelines and of patients for whom PCT-supported individual treatment was carried out according to the algorithms specified in Figure 6.3 (23).

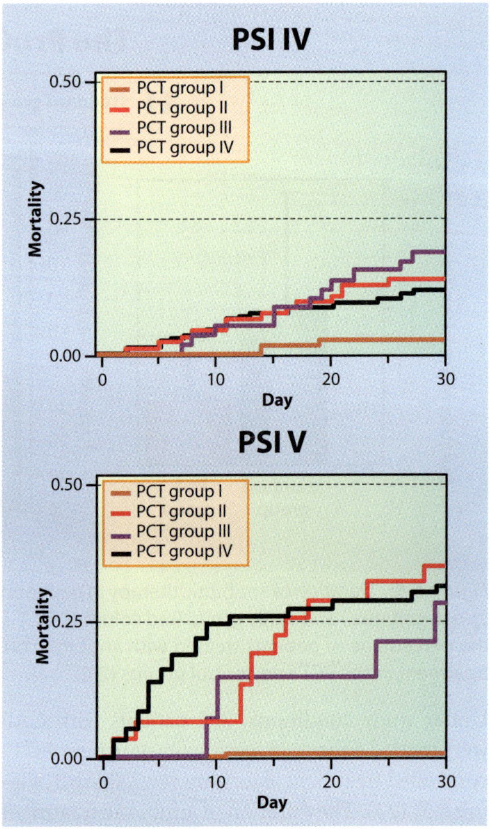

Figure 6.8: Mortality risk of community-acquired pneumonia of differing levels of severity in patients with normal PCT levels (group 1) and elevated PCT levels. PSI = Pulmonary Severity Index.
Group 1: PCT <0.1 ng/ml, Group 2: PCT 0.1-0.25 ng/ml. Group 3 PCT 0.25-0.5 ng/ml. Group 4 PCT >0.5 ng/ml (35).

6.3. Control of antibiotic treatment in patients in intensive care with sepsis, severe sepsis and septic shock

In intensive care, PCT monitoring can also help adapt the duration of treatment with antibiotics individually to the requirements of patients. This generally leads to a reduction in the length of antibiotic treatment cycles.

▶ Patients with severe sepsis or septic shock

In a study by Nobre et al., the duration of treatment with antibiotic in the PCT-controlled patient group with severe sepsis or septic shock – regardless of the cause of the illness – was shorter than for patients in the control group by up to 4 days (☞ Figure 6.9) (25). The different in patients treated "per protocol" was 4 days (6 vs. 10 days), and in the "intention to treat" group it was 3.5 days. Breaking of the rules was observed in 19% of patients, that is, the physicians did not follow the PCT-controlled algorithm. In patients with positive blood cultures, the difference was 6 days (13 vs. 7 days). In this study, besides the absolute value of the PCT levels, their progression was also evaluated (☞ Table 6.1). The rate of complications and relapses were comparable between the two groups.

In another study carried out by Schroeder and Hochreiter et al., the example of a smaller group of patients with severe sepsis (n = 27) was used, with a PCT-controlled treatment algorithm, to report a shorter duration of therapy by 1.7 days (8.3 ± 0.7 vs. 6.6 ± 1.1 days on average ± SD) in the PCT group (☞ Table 6.1) (369).

These studies show that an individual, patient-adapted antibiotic treatment using PCT is also possible for patients in intensive care.

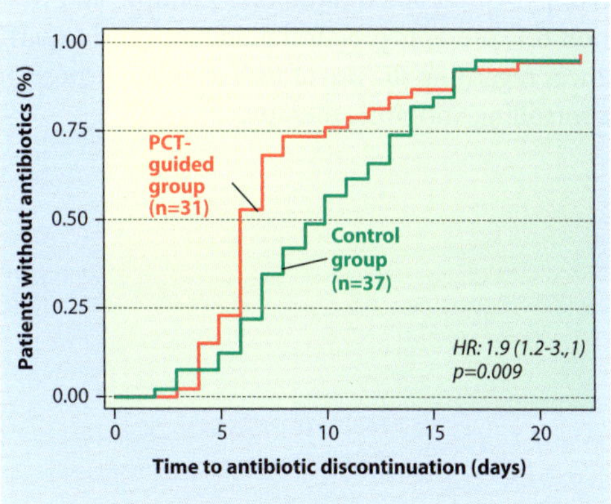

Figure 6.9: Number of patients in intensive care without antibiotic treatment in comparison with the control group (no PCT-controlled therapy) and intervention group (PCT-controlled treatment algorithm) (25). Duration of treatment of more than 6 to 8 days is obviously not necessary for certain patients.

In patients with at least two positive signs of SIRS and suspicion of infection (sepsis) in a surgical intensive care unit, a PCT-controlled treatment with antibiotic was carried out in comparison with a control group (356). When the clinical signs and symptoms of infection improved and PCT levels decreased to less than 1 ng/ml, antibiotic treatment was discontinued in the PCT group. Alternatively, the therapy was discontinued when the PCT level was still above 1 ng/ml, but had fallen after 3 days to less than 25 to 35% of its initial value. In this study, too, the duration of treatment with antibiotics in the PCT group, at 5.9 ± 1.7 days, was significantly shorter than the duration of treatment in the control group (7.9 ± 0.5 days of antibiotics) (☞ Table 6.1).

In clinical practice, the decision must be made in each case as to what limit values and PCT trends should be used to control or discontinue antibiotic therapy. Knowledge of the individual circumstances and the clinical experience of the treating physician increase the diagnostic reliability of the decision in the specific case (☞ Figure 1.6).

This has been highlighted by another study conducted in 630 intensive care patients [389]. In this study, a PCT-guided treatment algorithm in various infections also significantly reduced exposure to antibiotics compared with a control group, without any increase in mortality or increased re-infection rates.

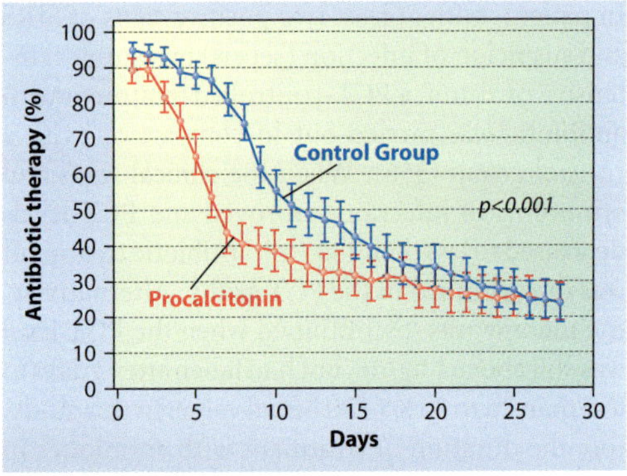

Figure 6.10: The "PRORATA" trial: Percent of patients receiving antibiotic therapy after acute onset of infection in the ICU, requiring immediate antibiotic therapy (septic shock, purulent meningitis etc.) (i) when treated according to general guidelines (blue line, no algorithm, n=319) or (ii) according to PCT values and clinical data (red line, PCT-guided algorithm, n=311, $p<0.001$) (389). The PCT-guided algorithm to support decisions to initiate antibiotic therapy was: PCT <0.25 ng/ml (or 0.25-0.5 ng/ml), antibiotics strongly disencouraged (disencouraged, respectively); PCT ≥0.5 ng/ml to <1 ng/ml, (≥1 ng/ml), antibiotics encouraged (strongly encouraged, respectively). The recommendation was to obtain a second PCT measurement 6-12 hours later, if the first measurement was obtained early after start of the episode. The PCT-guided algorithm to support decisions to stop, change or continue antibiotic therapy according to daily measured PCT values were: If PCT <0.25 ng/ml stop of antibiotics strongly recommended; if PCT ≥0.25 ng/ml to <0.5 ng/ml or decline of PCT more than 80% of previous PCT peak value: Stop of antibiotics recommended. If PCT values were ≥0.5ng/ml or decline was less than 80% decline of peak value: Continuation of antibiotics was recommended. If there was an increase of PCT value as compared to the previous maximum PCT values or if PCT was ≥0,5 ng/ml: Changing of antibiotics was strongly recommended (☞ Table 6.2).

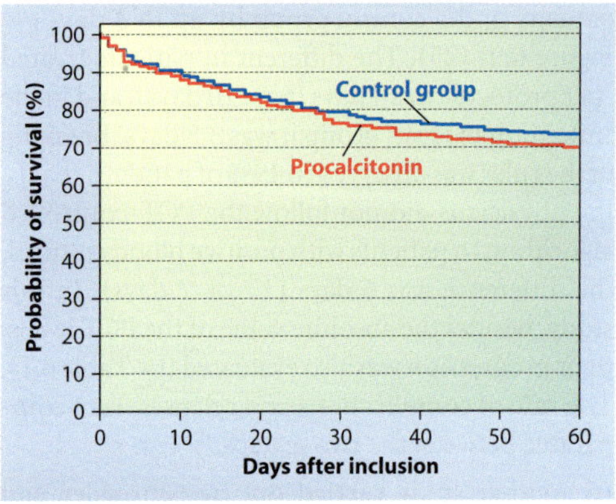

Figure 6.11: The survival rate on day 28 (and 60) was not significantly different among groups. Hence, the PCT guided algorithm did not harm the patients (OR day 28 0.82, IC 90% 0.56-1.20; OR day 60 1.02, IC 90% 0.72-1.45). Blue line, control group, no algorithm and conventional, guideline related antibiotic therapy. Red line, Procaclitonin-guided group with algorithm. P=0.31 by the log-rank test (389).

Since there is no generally valid data as to the treatment algorithm to be used in any specific case, Table 6.2 shows the theoretical basis for an individual, patient-adapted antibiotic therapy, and Section 6.1. presents practical guidelines and experiences regarding the use of PCT for the purpose of controlling antibiotic therapy.

7. Use for special indications

7.1. Diagnostic use of PCT in patients with pneumonia

▶ Community-acquired and nosocomial pneumonia ("CAP" and "HAP")

Pneumonia can occur in different forms and degrees of severity. Pneumonias are classified into different types depending on the cause and type of agent. The usual division is into "community-acquired pneumonia" (CAP) and "nosocomial pneumonia" (or "hospital-acquired pneumonia"). These differ in the range of agents and have different risks. "Ventilator-associated pneumonia" (VAP) can be seen as a limiting case of nosocomial pneumonia, which can occur 48 to 72 hours after intubation or mechanical ventilation (160). Moreover, pneumonias can also be classified by the type of agent. Examples are pneumonias caused by tuberculosis, fungal infection, atypical agents, or viral infections.

The diagnosis of a pneumonia is always a clinical diagnosis. It is based on the following three pillars:

1. Detection or suspicion of an infection of the airways (e.g. suppurative secretions, microbial findings in the tracheal secretions or bronchioalveolar lavage (BAL))

2. Signs of systemic inflammation (fever, leukocytosis, possible increase in other inflammation markers, e.g. CRP or PCT)

3. Indications of involvement of pulmonary parenchyma (e.g. infiltrates in the X-rays or CT).

The diagnosis of a pneumonia is primarily a clinical diagnosis.

Although a systemic inflammatory response occurs in pneumonia, PCT need not always be elevated (☞ Figure 7.1). The PCT levels measured in pneumonia may therefore be very different, even for bacterial pneumonia (☞ Figures 7.2a and 7.2b) (101, 102, 110, 111, 164, 172, 18, 36, 165, 167, 172, 173, 357).

There is sometimes a relationship to the mortality risk of the disease; in different studies of community-acquired pneumonia, very low PCT values characterized patients with low mortality (35, 357).

The induction of PCT depends on many factors: the type of agent, the severity of the pneumonia, and the degree of systemic inflammatory response.

Generally, PCT values for bacterial agents are higher than those for viral pneumonias, atypical agents (except for legionella pneumonia), or tuberculosis, where the induction of PCT is often absent or very slight.

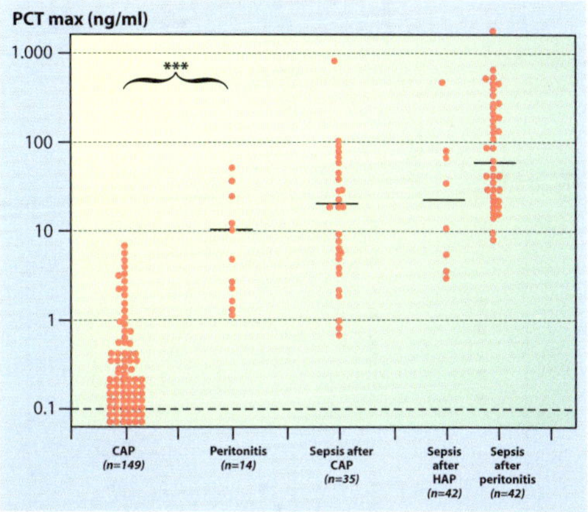

Figure 7.1: PCT serum concentration in pneumonia or peritonitis, with or without septic symptoms (maximum levels). The bars represent the median of each group. The pneumonia and peritonitis groups (columns 1 and 2) differ significantly (Mann-Whitney test p<0.001) (155).
CAP = Community acquired pneumonia; HAP = hospital acquired pneumonia.

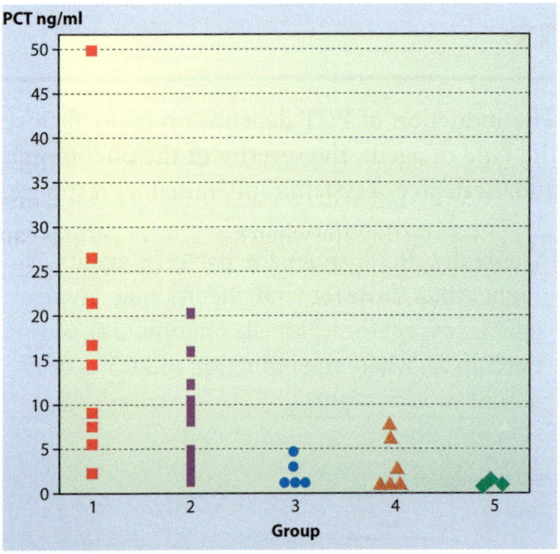

a

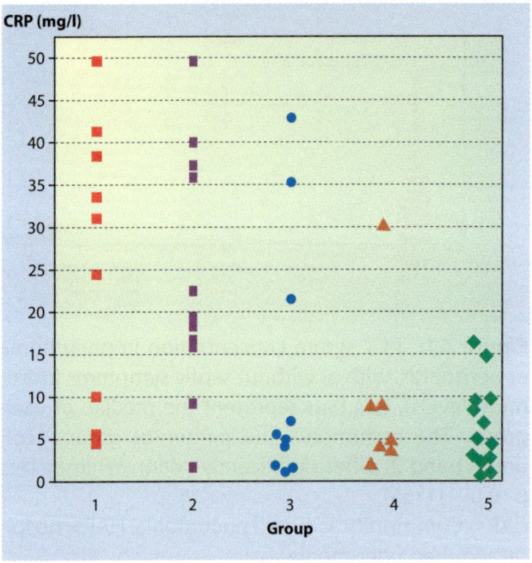

b

Figures 7.2a+b: PCT **(a)** and CRP **(b)** in children with community-acquired pneumonia with different causes. Groups 1 and 2: bacterial pneumonia (group 1, culture detection of *Streptococcus pneumoniae;* group 2, detection of *S. pneumoniae* in blood culture or sputum, including one patient with *Hemophilus influenzae b*, marked as Hib); group 3, mycoplasma, serologically positive test for *Mycoplasma pneumoniae;* groups 4 and 5, detection of virus: detection of viral agents (serological evidence, immunofluorescence, or culture) (group 4) or viral agent with bacterial superinfection (group 5) (102).

In viral pneumonias or pneumonias due to atypical agents such as chlamydia or mycoplasmas, elevated PCT levels are the exception, while for bacterial pneumonias or legionella pneumonia, elevated PCT levels can be observed in the majority of patients (101, 102, 161-166, 358) (☞ Figures 7.2a+b).

In tuberculosis, PCT induction also depends on the activity and the severity of the disease. In chronic illnesses, no significant induction of PCT can generally be expected. Induction can be very variable, however. There are reports of only slightly elevated PCT values of 0.3 ng/ml to around 1 ng/ml in active pulmonary tuberculosis from several authors (160-170). The PCT concentration in patients with pleural effusion in tuberculosis were also in a low range (0.1-0.3 ng/ml) (171). In one study of acute pneumonia in tuberculosis, the PCT value was elevated to 4.16 ng/ml (161).

A normal or only slightly elevated PCT value does not exclude the diagnosis of a bacterial pneumonia.

In some studies – depending on the patient population observed and the severity of the pneumonia – up to every second patient had PCT levels below the limit value of 0.5 ng/ml important in the diagnosis of sepsis (35, 357). In a study by Huang et al. (Pittsburgh), 28% of all patients accepted in the study with pneumonia had PCT values below 0.1 ng/ml. The tendency was observed that low PCT levels occurred more frequently in less severe pneumonia (PSI I to II). However, even patients with high risk profiles and bacterial pneumonia had low to normal PCT levels. It was noted, however, that despite a high "Pneumonia Severity Index" (PSI), which describes an elevated mortality risk, these patients had a significantly better prognosis than that described by the score (☞ Figure 6.8) (35). A study by Krüger et al. reached similar results. Here, too, patients with low PCT levels had a low mortality risk (357).

In pneumonia, PCT levels and their progression can provide important indications of the risk and progression of the disease.

For elevated PCT levels, pneumonia should always be considered (especially a bacterial pneumonia), while conversely, normal PCT levels cannot exclude a diagnosis of pneumonia. If there is pneumonia, observation of the progression of PCT levels is recommended in order to evaluate risk and monitor the success of therapy.

PCT levels can provide an information for treatment

PCT has been used in patients with community-acquired pneumonia to adapt the treatment indication and duration of treatment to the individual situation of the patient (☞ Section 6.2.5.). Just as procalcitonin is used for patients suspected of airway infections or patients with exacerbated COPD as an indication of the necessity of antibiotic treatment, in community-acquired pneumonia the PCT levels can also provide indications for the continuation or discontinuation of antibiotic treatment – if other clinical data is also integrated into the evaluation of the patient (☞ Section 6.2.3.). In some studies, the duration of treatment with antibiotics could be significantly reduced by using a PCT-controlled treatment algorithm for patients with pneumonia or sepsis, in comparison with patients without immune monitoring (22-24, 385, 389).

Moreover, in addition to the absolute value of the PCT levels, their progression is also significant. In different studies, decreasing PCT levels in patients with VAP were an indication of a good prognosis, and therefore the effectiveness of therapy (18, 20, 36, 174, 371). It therefore seems possible to use progression monitoring of PCT to achieve a reduction in the duration of antibiotic treatment even in patients with VAP, or to distinguish between therapy responders and "non-responders" (154, 158) (☞ Sections 6.2.5. and 6.3.).

PCT can be used diagnostically in pneumonias for the following reasons

- An elevated PCT level indicates a higher probability of the presence of a bacterial pneumonia or a higher severity of the disease (e.g. pneumonia with sepsis).
- Low PCT levels (under 0.1 ng/ml) occur more often in less severe pneumonias or those with low mortality risk to the patient, or in pneumonias with viral or atypical agents. They can be an indication that an antibiotic treatment may be unnecessary or no longer necessary.
- High PCT levels have been found more frequently in patients with ARDS due to bacterial causes, or with aspiration pneumonia, while in ARDS with non-bacterial causes the PCT levels were comparatively low, at least at the onset of the disease (175).
- The level and progression of PCT levels can provide information about the success of therapy, as well as the prognosis for the disease. Under some circumstances, this information can be used to control therapy (e.g. switching antibiotics if the PCT levels fail to decrease within a few days; discontinuing therapy when no more infiltrates can be detected and the PCT levels have decreased below a certain range of concentrations).

7.2. Bacteremia

In patients with positive blood cultures, PCT levels are often higher than in patients with the same disease in whom no germs can be found in the blood. These patients usually also have a particularly severe progression or a poorer prognosis (sepsis, pneumonia, endocarditis, oncological diseases) (23, 176-178).

Very low PCT levels, on the other hand, have a high negative predictive value for the exclusion of bacteremia (☞ Table 7.1). PCT is thus often elevated when there is evidence of bacterial agents in the blood ("bacteremia"). A correlation of microbiological findings ("positive blood cultures") with PCT levels is impractical in the absence of knowledge of the patient and the clinical relationships, since the term "bacteremia" alone describes the presence of bacterial agents in the circulating blood without describing the reaction of the body to those agent. PCT, on the other hand, describes the inflammatory and immunological reaction of the organism to the corresponding agents or inflammatory situations. Thus, in sepsis PCT levels are on an average higher in patients with positive blood cultures, and positive blood cultures are more frequently seen in patients with high PCT levels or severe sepsis or those with severe organ dysfunction (3). If the inflammatory response is weak or only temporary, PCT may not be elevated, even if the blood culture is positive.

A lack of reaction by the organism and therefore a low PCT level may also contribute to evaluation of contamination of the blood with coagulase-negative staphylococcus. For contamination with this bacterium, PCT levels have been shown to be significantly lower than in bacteremia. At a limit value of 0.1 ng/ml, PCT had a sensitivity of 100% and a specificity of 80% for the diagnosis of a bacteremia on the day of admission. PCT levels on

Cut-off	Sensitivity	Negative predictive value	AUC	Literature, number of patients
3.03 ng/ml	83%	83%	0.80	(178), n=33 (12 with bacteremia)
0.5 ng/ml 0.2 ng/ml	57% (31-84)* 93 (79-100)*	92 (86-98)* 97 (92-100)*	0.7	(180), n=108 (14 with bacteremia)
1.0 ng/ml	63.8%	96.8%	n.a.	(177), n=107 (11 with bacteremia)
0.5 ng/ml 0.2 ng/ml	56% 92%	96% 99%		(181), n=200 (50 with bacteremia)
0.4 ng/ml	95.2%	98.8%	0.83	(182), n=165 (22 with bacteremia)
1.9 ng/ml <0.5 ng/ml	80% 100%	n.a.	0.84	(183), n=29 (13 with bacteremia)
1.1 ng/ml	57%	92%	0.76	(184), n=103 (12 patients with gram-neg. bacteremia, patients with neutropenia and leukemia)
0.5 ng/ml	58%	87%	0.71	(185), n=78 (20 with bacteremia; neutropenic patients, time 0 to 10 hours)
0.5 ng/ml	66.7%	93.9%	n.a.	(186), n=87 (10 with bacteremia, neutropenic patients after chemotherapy)
2.45 ng/ml	n.a.	96%	n.a.	(179), n=300 (new onset of fever, Internal Medicine)
2.0 ng/ml	57%	98%	n.a.	(187) (215 children 3 to 36 months old, fever)

Table 7.1: Sensitivity and negative predictive value (NPV) of a bacteremia using PCT. *95% confidence interval. AUC = area under the curve of the sensitivity/specificity diagram.

the day before release and the day after release were also significant (377). In this study, even for bacteremia, the measured PCT levels were in a low range (on average, 0.5 to 0.6 ng/ml), that a limit value of < 0.1 to 0.2 ng/ml is important here as well.

If the "risk" of presence of a bacteremia is to be evaluated using PCT, high PCT levels (e.g. PCT >2.4 ng/ml (179)) are an important indication of possible bacteremia with systemic inflammatory response, the accuracy of which can be improved by considering additional factors (e.g. temperature, albumin, leukocyte, or thrombocyte levels) in the context of a decision tree ("Classification and Regression Tree" or "CART analysis") (179)). In the decision tree developed by Peters et al. to predict bacteremia, PCT is the most important discriminator in patients with fever (179).

Conversely, patients with very low PCT (<0.2 ng/ml) often have negative blood cultures. The high sensitivity and high negative predictive value of very low PCT levels can therefore be used diagnostically for the exclusion of bacteremia, as can the higher probability of positive blood cultures for high PCT levels (the negative predictive value of PCT to exclude bacteremia for PCT levels below 0.1 to 0.5 ng/ml is in the range from 87 to 99%) (☞ Table 7.1). The result for a positive blood culture (specificity, positive predictive value), however, depends strongly on the reasons for elevated PCT in individual patients or in the population examined, thus the so-called "pretest probability" (e.g. sepsis of various causes). The specificity of the marker for the diagnosis of bacteremia is thus not included in Table 7.1.

For very low PCT levels, the presence of bacteremia is improbable.

7.3. Bacterial endocarditis

PCT is often elevated in patients with endocarditis. Despite its relative high sensitivity, PCT is not the gold standard for the diagnosis of endocarditis (☞ Table 7.2). That is generally echocardiography. However, there are patients for whom the diagnosis of endocarditis has been found on the basis of elevated PCT levels. Even echocardiography can

PCT (ng/ml) endocarditis	PCT (ng/ml) control group	Sensitivity, specificity; PPV, NPV	Number of patients observed	Literature
6.56 (median)	0,44	81%, 85%; 72%, 92%, cut-off 2.3 ng/ml	21 patients with confirmed bacterial endocarditis out of a total of 67 patients examined	(190)
0.12 ± 0.13 (average ± SD) (range 0-0.4 ng/ml)	< detection limit		30 patients with endocarditis without sepsis and 20 controls	(189)
3.48 ng/ml PCT level on admission (median)	0.19 ng/ml	100%, 93%; 92%, 100%	50 patients with bacterial endocarditis and 50 healthy controls	(191)

Table 7.2: PCT levels in patients with endocarditis. Diagnosis is generally made based on the Duke criteria. These include two "major" criteria (transesophageal echo, blood culture) and five "minor" criteria (fever, predisposing illness, blood vessel anomalies, immunological changes, and at least three positive serological microbial findings). For the diagnosis, either 2 major and 1 minor criteria, or 1 major and 3 minor criteria are necessary; PPV and NPV are positive and negative predictive value, respectively.

provide false-negative results in some cases in the beginning stages of the disease (including transesophageal echocardiography, TEE). There are case reports of patients with initially negative TEE findings and atypical clinical symptoms who exhibited elevated PCT levels, which days later led to an echocardiographically substantiated diagnosis of endocarditis. However, it is more frequent in the everyday clinical routine for patients with endocarditis to have very nonspecific symptoms at first, and for these not to be recognized as signs of infection in a timely manner. With elevated PCT levels and nonspecific clinical symptoms (e.g. circulatory problems, nonspecific changes in consciousness like somnolence, focal blackouts, fever, shivering, etc.), bacterial endocarditis should always be considered during the search for the focus, particularly if cardiac risk factors are present (heart valve defect, heart valve replacement, weakened immunity, intravenous drug abuse) (188). Naturally, there are also patients with endocarditis and unremarkable PCT levels, for example in the absence of a systemic inflammatory response (189).

Bacterial endocarditis can be overlooked in the context of acute diagnostics, because the general symptoms are often nonspecific and echocardiography is not done. In rare cases, the disease may be missed even by echocardiography in its early stages.

An elevated PCT level has already indicated a diagnosis of endocarditis in numerous patients. Elevated PCT levels with appropriate symptoms should therefore always be reason to consider endocarditis, even though the marker need not be elevated in every patient with endocarditis.

The optimum cut-off value for the diagnosis of endocarditis has been given as 2 to 3 ng/ml in various studies. However, a significantly lower limit value should be used to exclude endocarditis (0.1 ng/ml to 0.25 ng/ml).

The results of studies of bacterial endocarditis and PCT are summarized in Table 7.2.

7.4. Acute bacterial meningitis

Acute bacterial meningitis is always life-threatening. Early diagnosis and effective antibiotic therapy are decisive for the progression and prognosis of the disease.

Routine diagnostic data, including cerebrospinal fluid puncture, do not always permit an immediate, clear diagnosis (☞ Table 7.3). Here, PCT can offer additional safety, since high PCT levels in the plasma in conjunction with appropriate clinical symptoms indicate bacterial meningitis or sepsis

	Number of patients	Acute bacterial meningitis	Viral meningitis	Sensitivity/specificity (cut-off value); positive and negative predictive value (PPV/NPV)	Literature
PCT (ng/ml) (average ± SD) CRP (mg/l) Cell count (/µl) Protein content (g/l)	59, children	54.5 + 35.1 (4,8-110) 144.1 + 69.1 (28-311) 5156 + 4336 (250-17500) 2.3 + 1.2 (0.4-4.7) (18 pat.)	0.32 + 0.35 (0-1.7) 14.8 + 14.1 (0-48) 390 + 648 (20-3200) 0.62 + 0.47 (20-3200) (41 pat.)	94%/100% (5 ng/ml)	(99)
PCT (average, range) CRP	30, adults	1.75 (0.16-59.9) 174 (7-400)	0.24 (0.12-0.29) 7 (2-65)	69%/100% (0.5 ng/ml) 100%/74% 94%/57% (8mg/l)	(193)
PCT (average, range) CRP	45, adults	6.45 (0.25-43.776) 152 (25-367)	0.27 (0.05-0.44) 8 (3-78)	90%/100% (0.5 ng/ml) 100%/93% 90%/92% (50 mg/l); 90%/92%	(196)
PCT (average, range) CSF protein	167, children	9.1 (0.2-107) 1.4 (0.4-5.3)	0.2 (0.1-4.4) (aseptic meningitis) 0.4 (0.1-1.8)	89%/89% (0.5 ng/ml) 86%/78% (0.5 g/l);	(192)
PCT (median, 95% percentile) CRP Cell count (leukocytes)	151, adults	2.45 (0.7-3.7) 162 (39-275) 494 (204-1300)	0.07 (0-0.08) non-bact. meningitis) 13 (9-17) 98 (70-127)	87%/100% (2.13 ng/ml) 100%/ 99% (PPV/NPV) 78%/74% (22 mg/l) 28%/96% (PPV/NPV 50%/94% (300 /mm^3) 53%/94% (PPV/NPV)	(194)

Table 7.3: Serum levels of PCT (ng/ml) and CRP (mg/l), cell count, and protein content of the cerebrospinal fluid in patients with acute bacterial or viral meningitis. If not otherwise specified, the values shown represent the average ± standard deviation from the average, along with the range of values measured.

with high probability, while for normal or low PCT levels both diagnoses are improbable (99, 109, 192-194). For viral meningitis, PCT levels are usually barely elevated. For bacterial meningitis, PCT levels are primarily above 0.5 ng/ml. One exception is local bacterial infection, e.g. infected cerebrospinal fluid drainages, which cannot be diagnosed reliably with PCT (195). PCT level measurement in the cerebrospinal fluid, unlike Interleukin-6, is ineffective, since PCT levels are often no higher than in the plasma and PCT in the cerebrospinal fluid can also not be measured reliability with the measurement methods routinely in use (109).

If there is clinical suspicion of meningitis, particularly for an elevated PCT level, antibiotic treatment should be started in any case. Since PCT can also provide no complete diagnostic reliability for the diagnosis or exclusion of bacterial or viral meningitis, if there are positive clinical symptoms it is recommended to start an initial antibiotic treatment even if the PCT level is negative. Over the course of the next day or two, if negative PCT levels persist and if bacterial meningitis is improbable due to other data, the treatment can be discontinued.

It was shown during a meningitis epidemic in France that this procedure is effective: daily PCT level measurement permitted significant reductions in the quantity of antibiotics prescribed and the duration of hospital care in comparison with an earlier epidemic (from 46% to 29%, and 4.5 to 2.1 days) 46% (34).

> If meningitis is suspected, PCT level measurement should be included in the standard diagnostic routine.

For patients with cerebrospinal fluid drainage (e.g. external ventricle drainage), on the other hand, PCT should not be used for infection monitoring (either in the cerebrospinal fluid or in the plasma). Since these are generally local bacterial infections, the sensitivity of the marker is very limited (195). Classical signs of infection in the cerebrospinal fluid, such as cell counts, glucose and lactate levels, and microbiological cultures are still the diagnostic standard for these cases.

PCT is also elevated in meningococcal infections. This disease progresses with great speed, and is associated with a high mortality risk. High PCT levels (e.g. >10 ng/ml) indicate a high risk of death and a high risk for organ dysfunction (☞ Section 9.3.) (381, 382). PCT can improve diagnostics in this case, as well. There are false-negative results, so that even for a negative PCT level with clinical suspicion of meningococcal infection, a treatment should be started immediately, but the high sensitivity of PCT still improves diagnostics, since conventional diagnostics also provide false-negative findings. Patients have fallen ill or died even with a negative cerebrospinal fluid finding. Elevated PCT levels are thus an additional indication for the presence of a severe bacterial disease. This is particularly important during a meningococcus epidemic (381).

7.5. Differential diagnosis of viral diseases

PCT is generally not induced, or is induced only in small amounts, in viral diseases. Numerous studies support this statement. This doesn't necessarily mean that a measurable increase in PCT cannot occur in individual cases or severe disease progression. A concentration range from 1 to 2 ng/ml, however, is only seldom exceeded. In 274 children with viral infections, the average PCT level was 0.39 ± 0.57 ng/ml. Only 16 children had values over 1 ng/ml (specificity 94%) (197). The following diseases were examined: meningitis with enterovirus, tick encephalitis, pneumonias due to parainfluenza, adenovirus, influenza, or RS virus, diarrhea from rotavirus, and systemic viral diseases from influenza, RS, parainfluenza, adeno-, or herpes simplex viruses, and viral hepatitis (☞ Figure 7.3).

In comparison with CRP, PCT has a higher sensitivity and specificity for the differential diagnosis of bacterial and viral infections (41).

There is additional data supporting low induction of PCT in viral diseases:

Resch et al. studied children with diseases of the airways and RSV-positive bronchiolitis (aged less than one year, 31 children). The PCT level in all children was less than 0.5 ng/ml (112). Similar results were found in Epstein-Barr virus infections: 23 of 25 children had PCT levels under 0.5 ng/ml. CRP, on the other hand, was less than 10 mg/l in only 7 children (limit value for the diagnosis of bacterial infections); 5 children had levels above

40 mg/l (49 to 176 mg/l) (198). Classical signs of infection were unhelpful for a differential diagnosis: 50% of children had leukocytosis, 25% an elevated BSG (>30 mm/h).

Other data has been obtained from comparative studies of bacterial and viral infections in meningitis (34, 99, 106, 193) or pneumonia (102, 110, 111, 164, 165) (☞ Sections 7.3. and 8.2.) as well as in tick encephalitis (199).

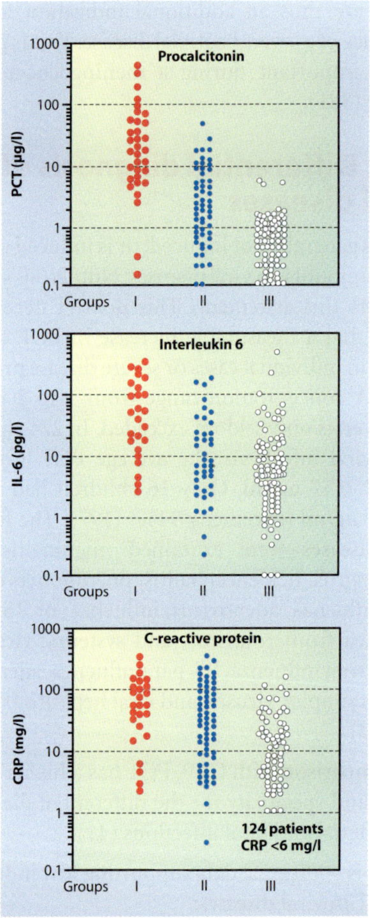

Figure 7.3: Comparison of serum concentrations of PCT, CRP, and IL-6 in children with invasive bacterial infections (Group I), local bacterial infection (Group II), and viral infection (Group III). Group I: 53 children (aged 2.3 years on average) with positive blood culture (n=31) or bacterial meningitis. Group II: 109 children with local bacterial infections (negative blood culture, also pneumonia; aged 4.2 years on average). Group III: 274 children with viral illnesses (viral evidence) (aged 2.3 years on average) (197).

There is also data for the lung disease SARS. Two patients had PCT levels of 0.1 ng/ml and 0.74 ng/ml despite bilateral pulmonary infiltrates (113). For H5N1 avian flu, there has been no data published to date. PCT levels here may be somewhat higher, since there is massive production of proinflammatory cytokines. In HIV-1 infection, PCT is also not significantly elevated (114). Additional data on viral diseases and PCT has been published by Delevaux et al. (200). Median levels were 0.2 ng/ml (range 0.1-1.1 ng/ml), with CPR levels at 15 mg/l (1.9-145 mg/l).

In viral hepatitis, mildly elevated PCT levels occur (range 0.5 to 1 ng/ml) (201).

PCT can therefore provide indications of viral and bacterial causes for a disease when there are signs of inflammation, if these alternatives are diagnostically suspected.

7.6. Fungal diseases: Aspergillus and candida infections

Invasive fungal diseases can induce PCT in advanced stages (8, 202, 203). PCT is rarely induced in local fungal infections or less severe illness, however. But even for severe fungal infections there are cases in which the induction of PCT is low or nonexistent (7, 9, 10). Immune suppression or neutropenia can also lead to a reduced PCT reaction in fungal diseases (7).

In fungal infections, the peak value is only achieved on the third to fifth day of the disease, sometimes later (11, 202, 204, 205). Elevated PCT levels are an indication of a poor prognosis or an advanced stage of the disease (205).

If antibiotic treatment is unsuccessful and PCT levels continue elevated or increasing, invasive fungal disease should be considered (11, 206). Since PCT is not a specific marker, PCT levels are not an indication whether there is a fungal infection or not. However, there is still some information about the PCT levels that typically occur in fungal infections: In a study by Charles et al., the median PCT levels in bacteremia were 9.7 ng/ml, while in patients with candidemia it was often lower: here, concentrations of 0.1 to 5.5 ng/ml were more often measured in the serum (median 0.6 ng/ml). The typical diagnostic upper limit in this study was specified as 5.5 ng/ml (10).

If PCT is elevated in a fungal infection, the progression often correlates with the success of therapy: for successful therapy, the plasma level for many patients decreased more quickly than for bacterial diseases, while in other patients it at least did not continue to increase (8, 205, 206).

Fungal diseases should not primarily be diagnosed using PCT. Persistently elevated or increasing PCT levels, however, can indicate a fungal infection. The PCT level need not be very high in this case.
Particularly for protracted disease progression in intensive care, the possibility of a fungal infection should be considered if the PCT level does not return to the normal range after antibiotic treatment.

7.7. Autoimmune diseases

Autoimmune diseases generally induce little to no PCT. Reports from different working groups have confirmed this in more than 200 patients. In some forms of autoimmune diseases, however, there may be an increase in PCT, although levels of 1 or 2 ng/ml are only exceeded in a few special diseases (☞ Figures 5.1 and 7.4).

▶ Autoimmune diseases generally induce no PCT, however, there are exceptions

One exception is Wegener's granulatoma or anti-neutrophile cytoplasmatic antibody positive vasculitis (ANCA) and Goodpasture's Syndrome. PCT levels of more than 0.5 ng/ml, sometimes up to 3 ng/ml, have been described (100, 207, 208, 360). In Goodpasture's Syndrome, PCT levels of more than 100 ng/ml have been demonstrated in isolated cases (360). PCT values of over 0.5 ng/ml have also been observed in Kawasaki Syndrome and Still's Disease (116, 117, 197). An increase in PCT has been observed in children with autoimmune hepatitis and primary sclerosing cholangitis, while PCT was normal for toxic liver damage (363). The exact causes of increased PCT in these diseases are unclear, but adhesion or tissue invasion of immunocompetent cells or the release of proinflammatory cytokines could be the reason for the PCT induction. The adherence and tissue invasion of circulating leukocytary cells is an important step in the induction of PCT (☞ Section 4.3.).

In Kawasaki Syndrome, Goodpasture's Syndrome, Wegener's Disease, or anti-neutrophil antibody-positive vasculitis, mildly elevated or occasional significantly elevated PCT levels can be measured.

All other autoimmune diseases examined to date generally (that is, in 95% of cases) have PCT levels below the threshold for a sepsis diagnosis, 0.5 ng/ml. The median measured value was 0.2 ng/ml, although these concentrations were measured with techniques at their lower limit of measurement accuracy.

It is often asked whether immune suppression hinders the induction of PCT. Patients with autoimmune diseases frequently take immune suppressants. No significant suppression of PCT induction has been observed, aside from complete neutropenia, where induction can be limited by a third to a half in comparison with non-neutropenic patients (209, 210). Even patients with autoimmune diseases and infections had PCT levels of over 0.5 ng/ml (☞ Figures 5.1 and 7.4) (100). Even after organ transplantation, after which immune suppression is regularly done, many studies have shown a regular induction of PCT in sepsis and infections. The marker can therefore still be used for diagnosis of sepsis in autoimmune diseases and patients taking immune suppressants.

A diagnosis of infection and sepsis is possible with PCT even in autoimmune diseases and during immune suppression.

For the following autoimmune diseases, data on PCT is available: Wegener's granulomatosis or anti-neutrophil cytoplasmic antibody-positive vasculitis (ANCA), microscopic polyangitis (MPA), Goodpasture's Syndrome, Still's Disease, rheumatoid arthritis, juvenile chronic arthritis, systemic lupus erythematosus, different arthritides, ulcerative colitis, polymyositis, systemic sclerodermia, sarcoidosis, amyloidosis, thyreoiditis (100, 116, 117, 197, 200, 207, 208, 211-214, 360).

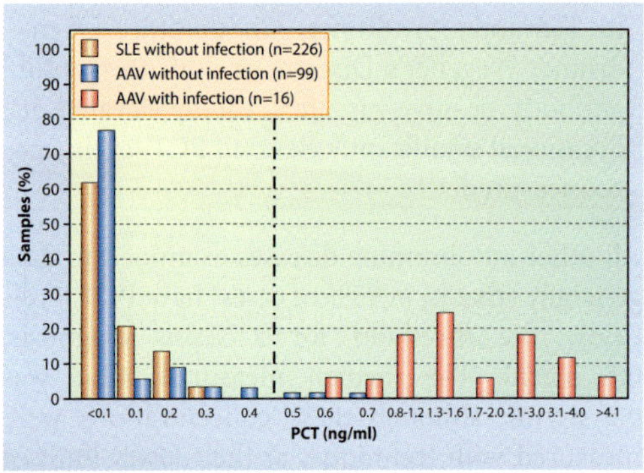

Figure 7.4: Distribution of average values of PCT serum samples from patients with systemic lupus erythematosis (SLE, 18 patients, all without infection) and with antineutrophil antibiotic-associated vasculitis (AAV, 35 patients), with and without bacterial infection (systemic infection, 16 patients). The values were measured in the early phase of the infection. The solid line denotes the reference range of PCT for non-septic disease (100).

7.8. Allergic diseases

Significant induction of PCT has not yet been described in allergic diseases.

7.9. Pancreatitis

The significance of PCT in the diagnosis of pancreatitis is often asked: can the marker distinguish between infected and non-infected necroses, indicate surgical operations or CT-controlled drainages, detect the severity or cause of pancreatitis, or indicate antibiotic therapy or CT examinations?

Of course, PCT cannot make these differentiations and decisions alone. However, the marker can indicate probabilistic tendencies for the evaluation of appropriate questions.

The available data on pancreatitis is variable. Some studies come to the conclusion that PCT can provide information to differentiate between infected and non-infected necroses, while others find only a correlation, often an early one, with the severity or prognosis of the disease. A meta-analysis accentu-

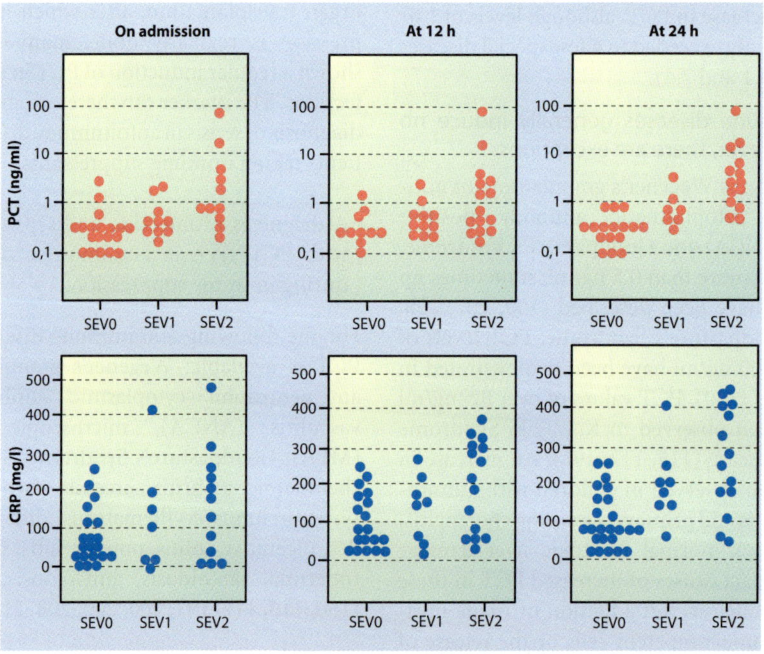

Figure 7.5: PCT and CRP levels in patients with acute pancreatitis. Distribution of severity according to Atlanta criteria, 1992 (218): SEV0, mild pancreatitis (n=30); SEV1, severe pancreatitis without organ dysfunction (n=11); SEV2, severe pancreatitis with organ dysfunction (n=16) (219). PCT can be used even at an early stage to obtain an indication of the severity of the disease: very low PCT levels are generally a sign of a mild severity of pancreatitis, while in prognostically unfavorable diseases high PCT levels occur with greater probability even in the early stages.

ates the fact that PCT can provide information both about the severity and the risk of bacterial infections in pancreatitis (215).

It is unarguable that the diagnostic value of PCT in these questions is significantly better than that of CRP.

Different studies have found a good correlation between PCT and the severity of pancreatitis. In mild pancreatitis or edematous pancreatitis, PCT levels are primarily low (under 0.5 to 0.8 ng/ml), while in severe pancreatitis it frequently exceeds 0.5 ng/ml. This particularly applies to early PCT level measurements, underscoring the prognostic properties of the marker. In different studies, PCT concurred with the Ranson score or the Atlanta system (☞ Figure 7.5).

In other studies, patients with infected necroses or mortality outcome had significantly higher values for PCT, but not for CRP, although the correlation with the severity of the disease was not unambiguously statistically confirmed in all studies (☞ Figures 7.6, 7.7a+b) (16, 104, 221). Only a few studies describe different data (222, 223).

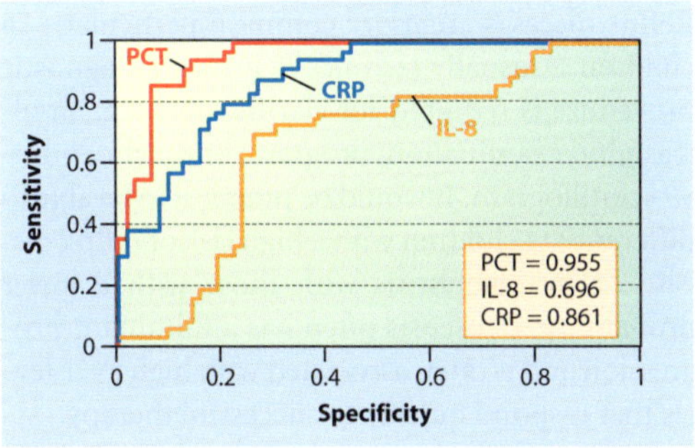

Figure 7.6: Sensitivity and specificity of PCT, CRP, and IL-8 for the diagnosis of infected necrosis. The area under the curve is 0.955 for PCT, 0.861 for CRP, and 0.696 for IL-8 (231).

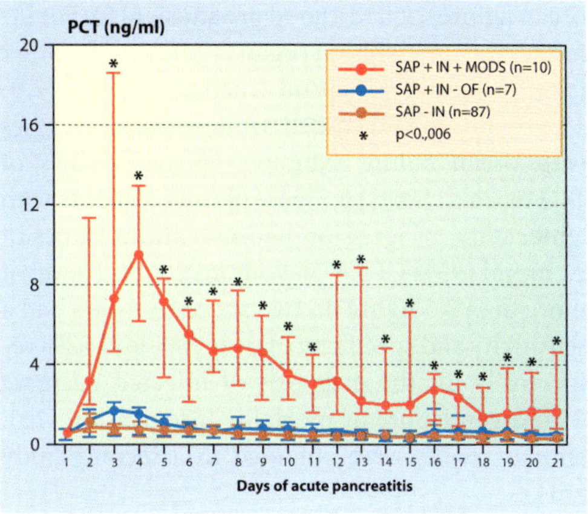

a

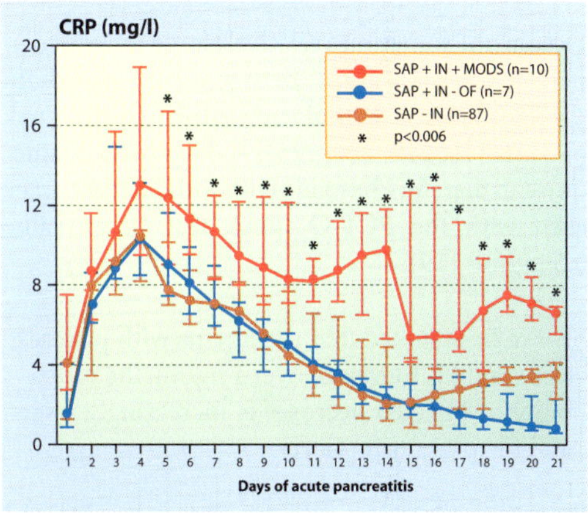

b

Figures 7.7a+b: PCT (☞ Figure 7.7a) and CRP (☞ Figure 7.7b) in severe acute pancreatitis (SAP) in patients with infected necroses (IN) with and without organ failure (MODS) (SAP+IN+MODS; SAP+IN-OF) and sterile necroses or edematous pancreatitis independent of organ failure (SAP-IN) (16).

> Essentially, higher PCT levels can be expected for severe pancreatitis, infected necroses and the occurrence of organ dysfunction than for patients with only a low severity of pancreatitis, no infection, and no organ dysfunction.
> The range of dispersion of the values can be large in some cases. Therapeutic decisions should therefore not be made based on the PCT levels alone.

In a multicenter study including 104 patients, the maximum median PCT levels were 1.4 ng/ml if the patient had no infected necroses (with or without organ failure) or had a good prognosis (16). For infected necroses without organ failure, on the other hand, values of 9.7 ng/ml (median, 95% CI 2.0-18.8 ng/ml) were recorded, while infected necroses with organ failure exhibited median values of 14.2 ng/ml (95% CI 8.7-54.2 ng/ml). Patients with a mortality progression had maximum values of 22 ng/ml (95% CI 5.6-56.9 ng/ml). A PCT level of more than 3.5 ng/ml on two successive days had a sensitivity and specificity of over 90% and 82% respectively for the diagnosis of infected necroses with organ failure or mortality progression (16). Similar results were obtained in a second study (104).

▶ What are the consequences of PCT level measurement in pancreatitis?

Despite the sometimes relatively large range of dispersion, limit values between 0.5 ng/ml to 1.4 ng/ml can be formulated to distinguish at-risk patients (16, 219, 224, 225). A diagnostic distinction can therefore be made with sufficient accuracy even with the PCT-Q quick test (limit value 0.5 ng/ml) (19).

> It can be assumed that in patients with pancreatitis and PCT levels of over 1 ng/ml, the probability of infected necroses is increasingly large and the prognosis poorer.

Prognostically useful data can already be obtained early in the disease progression. In various studies, high PCT levels as early as admission of the patient or in the first few days of the disease were already an indication of a poor prognosis or severe disease (104, 223, 225-227).

Low PCT levels, conversely, were more frequent in patients with good prognoses or without infection (high negative predictive value and high sensitivity of the marker for low limit values). A low PCT level therefore tends to contraindicate cost-intensive diagnostic and therapeutic measures such as repeated CT examinations, thin needle biopsies, or ongoing intensive care monitoring – even if prospective examinations or surgical studies have not yet been carried out in the case.

The question of necessity of antibiotic treatment depending on PCT levels has not yet been studied in pancreatitis. In principle, however, the prophylactic administration of highly effective antibiotic for pancreatitis is disputed – at least in mild forms of the disease, and possibly even for severe pancreatitis. Low PCT levels could be an indication of a lack of necessity of antibiotic therapy, while when the levels exceed certain limits values, an antibiotic treatment could be indicated. Prospective interventional studies must clarify this question, however.

Contrary to earlier reports, the cause of pancreatitis can be determined only poorly using PCT. One early study of patients with biliary pancreatitis found particularly high PCT levels, but subgroup analysis and studies by other working groups failed to confirm that data (219, 228-230).

7.10. Vesicourethral reflux, pyelonephritis, and urinary tract infections

Urinary tract infections are comparatively common. They are generally uncomplicated diseases. However, they can lead to kidney damage when they result in pyelonephritis and occur more frequently due to vesicourethral reflux. Pyelonephritis with sepsis can also result ("urosepsis"). Reflux diseases are more common particularly in children. A usually technically difficult diagnostic procedure is required for clarification, e.g. an ultrasound examination, urogram, or a technetium-99 scintillogram. It would be practical to be able to differentiate children with a high risk of reflux disease or pyelonephritis with those with a lower probability. Urosepsis often has a fulminant progression and is often associated with high PCT levels that respond quickly to successful therapy.

Children with changes to the renal pelvis (in the scintillogram) or vesicourethral reflux also have higher PCT levels on average than those with simple urinary tract infections (☞ Figure 7.8, Table 7.4). Conversely, children with normal PCT levels (e.g. PCT <0.25 ng/ml) hardly ever had severe reflux disease.

A high PCT level thus indicates a higher probability of the presence of pyelonephritis or vesicourethral reflux than a low PCT level (50, 51). The median PCT levels in reflux disease were 1.2 ng/ml, but without reflux 0.6 ng/ml. For a limit value of 0.5 ng/ml, the sensitivity for the diagnosis of a reflux disease was 85% (all stages) and 92% for a high-degree of reflux. The specificity of this find-

	Urinary tract infection (UTI)		Pyelonephritis		Number of patients (n); special notes Sensitivity, specificity, cut-off value, positive and negative predictive value (PPV/NPV)	Literature
	PCT (ng/ml)	CRP (mg/l)	PCT	CRP		
Pyelonephritis versus cystitis (average)	0,38 ± 0.19	30.3 ± 7.6	5.37 ± 1.9	120.8 ± 8.9	n=80; age: 1 month – 16 years Sensitivity/specificity for renal lesions: 70%/83% (PCT) 100%/26% (CRP)	(52)
Pyelonephritis versus control (median)	Control group: PCT 0.21 ng/ml (median)	51.4 mg/l	0.46 ng/ml (median)	220 mg/l No differences for WBC, BSR, fibrinogen	n=30 + 27 Sensitivity (0.5 ng/ml) and specificity: 44% and 92% (PCT); 94% and 33% (CRP)	(232)
Pyelonephritis versus UTI with fever (average)	0.44 ± 0.30	36.4 ± 26	4.48 ± 5.84	106 ± 68.8	n=100 Sensitivity (0.8 ng/ml) 83%, specificity 94% (PCT), PPV 94%, NPV 83%; 94%, 32%; PPV 61%, NPV 83% (CRP) Sensitivity of PCT for the prediction of renal changes in DMSA scintillography: 100%	(53)
Uuncomplicated UTI vs. Acute urinary tract infection with renal scarring (pyelonephritis) (median, 5/95 percentile)	0.31 (0.03-0.76)	7.20 (0-0.68)	9.28 (0.68-48.4) 1,16 for pyelonephritis	162 (0.0-350), 97 for pyelonephritis	n=77; children: aged 1 month – 12 years. Sensitivity 92%, specificity 62% (PCT, 1 ng/ml); 92%, 34% (CRP, 20 mg/l)	(163)
Acute pyelonephritis vs. UTI (median, range)	0.13 (0.02-2.15)	74.5 (14-235)	3.41 (0.36-12.4)	120 (8.2-26)	n=64; children: aged 2 weeks – 3 years. Sensitivity 94%, specificity 90% (PCT, 0.5 ng/ml); 100%, 18% (CRP, 20 mg/l)	(54)

Table 7.4: PCT and CRP in children with fever. Diagnosis of pyelonephritis or simple urinary tract infection.
WBC = leukocyte counts; BSR = blood sedimentation rate; CRP = C-reactive protein, UTI = urinary tract infection.

ing, however, was low. It was only 44%. 136 children were examined, aged 1 month to 4 years (median 9.7 months), of whom 25% had reflux (50). In a multicenter follow-up study including 398 children (of which again 25% had a reflux disease), these values were confirmed. The median PCT level was 1.6 ng/ml in reflux disease and 0.7 ng/ml without reflux. The sensitivity (limit 0.5 ng/ml) was 75% for all stages of the disease, and 100% for the diagnosis of more than a fourth-degree stage (51).

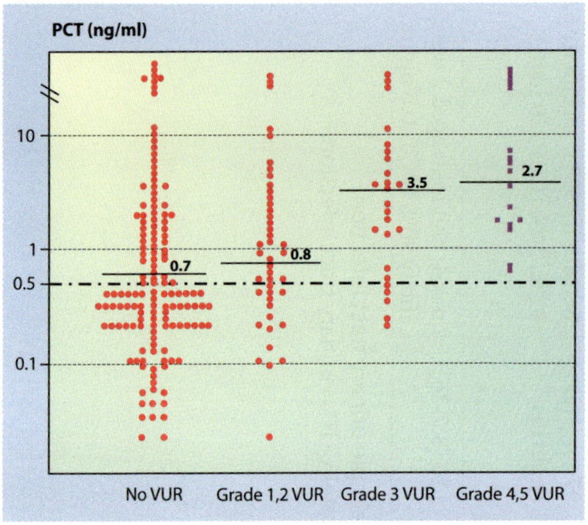

Figure 7.8: Distribution of PCT levels in children with different severity of vesicourethral reflux disease (VUR). The straight dotted line shows the median value for each group, while the solid line shows the limit value of 0.5 ng/ml (51). It is primarily the extreme values that are helpful for diagnosis: for a low PCT level of less than 0.2 ng/ml, the diagnosis of highly severe reflux is improbable, while for high levels the probability of diagnosis of a reflux disease increases.

One possible procedure would therefore be to omit further diagnostics for a negative PCT level (e.g. <0.1 ng/ml). For a high PCT level, however, it seems practical to start antibiotic treatment and introduce further pyelonephritis or reflux diagnostics at a higher urgency than for normal PCT levels.

8. Exceptions and special cases

8.1. PCT induction without indication of a bacterial focus

There are different situations in which PCT can be induced without evidence of bacterial infection (☞ Table 8.1). This may be the case, for example, in the first few days after severe trauma (accidental trauma, surgery, burns), during persistent circulatory shock, in multiple organ dysfunction, severe pancreatitis, or severe liver or kidney disease. In newborns, elevated PCT levels can be seen in the first few days after birth (☞ Chapter 9. and following).

Many factors can be possible reasons for a non-bacterial induction of PCT. For example, some that can be discussed as possible causes are tissue damage, high concentrations of proinflammatory cytokines in the plasma, or endotoxinemia as a consequence of intestinal underperfusion or bacterial translocation during problems with the barrier function of the intestines. Moreover, in rare cases there is paraneoplastic formation.

If high PCT levels occur without a bacterial cause, the problem is usually a severe disturbance of the homeostasis of the organism, or severe trauma. The risk that the immune system is affected and that there is thus a generally elevated risk of infection is high. In patients with greatly elevated PCT levels, even if no direct bacterial focus can be found, the continuation of antibiotic therapy can be a good idea.

Knowledge of the possible causes of non-bacterially induced PCT increases the diagnostic reliability

The non-bacterially induced formation of PCT has been observed:
• after surgery (☞ Section 8.2.)
• after severe trauma (polytrauma) (☞ Section 8.2.)
• after severe burns (☞ Section 8.1.)
• during prolonged cardiogenic shock (initially low, then increasing values in progression) (233-235)
• in severe perfusion problems, multiple organ failure, severe pancreatitis, possibly as the consequence of disturbances in intestinal microperforations and bacterial translocation
• during severe renal insufficiency and in patients with kidney replacement therapy (☞ Section 8.4.)
• in severe cirrhosis of the liver or acute or chronic viral hepatitis
• in newborns in the first few days of life (☞ Section 9.2.)
• after administration of anti-lymphocyte globulin, anti-CD3, or OKT-3 antibodies (without prior treatment with steroids) (☞ Sections 8.1. and 8.3.).
• in heat stroke (236, 237)
• in fungal infections (☞ Section 7.6.)
• in some autoimmune diseases (☞ Section 7.7.)
• after administration of higher doses of proinflammatory cytokines (238)
• in very rare cases of paraneoplastic, regularly in medullar or C-cell carcinoma (MCT) of the thyroid glands (239-241)
• in the end stages of severe tumor diseases (242) (☞ Section 8.5.)
• in some cases of severe rhabdomyolysis. Here, very PCT levels have sometimes been observed (236, 243, 244) (unpublished observations)
• after prolonged resuscitation, particularly with a poor prognosis (361, 362)
• in the very rarest of cases, for other reasons. Here, for example, cross-reactions and test antibodies must be ruled out (e.g. human antibodies to murine antibodies of the test system). Constant, highly elevated PCT levels indicate such (very rare) events.

Table 8.1: Diseases or conditions in which non-bacterially induced formation of PCT can occur.

of the interpretation of PCT in individual patients. One should therefore know these causes (☞ Table 8.1).

▶ Severe perfusion disorders, multiple organ dysfunction, pancreatitis

In persistent, severe multiple organ dysfunction, there is often a slight to medium increase in PCT, even if no direct bacterial focus can be detected. If the PCT levels of patients with organ dysfunction with and without infections are compared, at a comparable severity of organ dysfunction (e.g. the same SOFA score) patients with infections have significantly higher levels (☞ Figures 5.7 and 7.8) (6). We can observe a similar phenomenon in severe pancreatitis. Patients with pancreatitis and elevated PCT levels also generally have severe pancreatitis more frequently. Similarly, patients with infected necrosis had elevated PCT levels in numerous studies. But here, too, there are exceptions. In numerous patients, despite high PCT levels, no infected necrosis can be found (☞ Section 7.9, Figures 5.7 and 5.8). The clinical circumstances of the situation and the patient must therefore be taken into consideration in the individual case.

The cause of elevated PCT levels in multiple organ failure is unclear, just as in cardiogenic shock. It can be assumed that a bacterial translocation and intestinal barrier disorders, with subsequent endotoxinemia and systemic inflammatory response, play an important role. At least animal experiments support the idea that bacterial translocation occurs in perfusion disorders and pancreatitis. These may be at least partly responsible for PCT induction (222, 245).

▶ Prolonged cardiogenic shock

In severe cardiogenic shock, in addition to other inflammatory markers, PCT is also induced. At the onset of the disease, PCT levels are usually low, but they increase over the course of a severe disease requiring catecholamine (233). In contrast, in septic shock, at the onset of the disease PCT levels are usually high and with (successful) therapy they usually decrease rapidly.

De Werra reports PCT levels of 1.4 ng/ml on average in cardiogenic shock and much higher levels in septic shock (96 ng/ml, day 0 or 1 of diagnosis, average values) (233). Brunkhorst et al. also describe initially mildly elevated PCT levels in cardiogenic shock (also about 1.4 ng/ml), which then increase later with fever (to 33 ng/ml or more) (234). In studies by Geppert et al., patients with cardiogenic shock had PCT levels of about 0.8 ng/ml (median), but with septic shock about 9.2 ng/ml. After 13 hours, 25% of the patients with cardiogenic shock had PCT levels above 2 ng/ml (235).

Even in cardiogenic shock, if PCT levels are over 2 ng/ml one should think of bacterial sepsis; conversely, elevated PCT cannot exclude cardiogenic shock, especially if the poor circulatory condition has already persisted for a few days.

In patients with acute myocardial infarct, slightly elevated PCT levels have also been observed, even if there was no pump failure. This PCT increase, however, is relatively slight, and has hardly any differential diagnostic significance (243).

▶ Induction of PCT in renal insufficiency, hemodialysis, and hemofiltration

In severe renal insufficiency and some dialysis patients, basal slightly elevated PCT levels can be observed. More information on this can be found in Section 8.4..

▶ Severe cirrhosis of the liver and viral hepatitis

In patients with cirrhosis of the liver or acute or chronic viral hepatitis, we can also expect mildly elevated PCT levels (values around 0.5 to 1 ng/ml) (246, 247). In severe cirrhosis of the liver (Child C), some cases even exhibit elevated PCT levels of up to 4 ng/ml. This can make the diagnosis of a spontaneous bacterial peritonitis more difficult (363). In children with autoimmune hepatitis and primary sclerosing cholangitis, there are indications of elevated PCT levels (363).

▶ Induction of PCT after operations, trauma, transplantation

After operations, depending on the type and extent of the surgery, there may be a temporary induction of PCT. More details can be found in Section 8.2..

▶ Induction of PCT after resuscitation

After resuscitation, PCT levels may be elevated. Elevated PCT levels have particularly been reported after prolonged resuscitation and in patients with a poor prognosis (neurological outcome, pneumonia, mortality) (361, 362).

▶ PCT induction in severe burns and heat shock

After severe burns, inhalation trauma, and heat shock, regardless of infections, elevated PCT levels can be observed in the first few days (237, 248-251). Induction depends partly on the extent and severity of the burn (252, 253) or the inhalation trauma (252, 254-257). PCT has prognostic properties similar to a clinical scale, the "Unit Burn Standard" (UBS). The induction occurs early (that is, within 8 hours). It is not related to the presence of endotoxin (252). Other markers of inflammation are also induced after a burn trauma, e.g. interleukin-6 and CRP (249, 251, 257, 258). Measurement of progression and the interpretation of the absolute vale of the levels measured can help in some cases to differentiate between a possible sepsis and traumatically induced PCT, if the aforementioned restrictions are taken into consideration (259).

▶ Induction of PCT in tumor diseases

Induction of PCT in tumor diseases is rare. It can occur nonspecifically in the final stage of the disease, or – more rarely – paraneoplastically. Only in C-cell carcinoma of the thyroid gland are there regularly elevated calcitonin and PCT levels. Calcitonin and procalcitonin can be used in this case as a tumor marker. For more information on this topic, see Sections 8.5. and 8.6..

▶ PCT in autoimmune diseases

Although it is generally assumed that elevated PCT levels are not found in autoimmune diseases, specific autoimmune diseases have recently been observed with elevated PCT. More details can be found in Section 7.7..

▶ Induction in newborns in the first few days of life

In newborns within the first few days of life, there is nonspecific induction of different proinflammatory markers, including PCT (260-262) (☞ also Chapter 9. and following). The use of specific reference ranges for these first few days of life nevertheless allows PCT to be successfully used for the early diagnosis of sepsis and clinical decision-making.

▶ Elevated PCT levels in the elderly and in various non-inflammatory diseases

With low frequency (less than 7% of patients), older patients and patients with various non-inflammatory diseases exhibit PCT levels that are slightly above 0.1 ng/ml. A concentration of over 0.3 ng/ml, however, is achieved only seldom, so that this observation plays very little role in the diagnosis of sepsis (48).

▶ Induction by proinflammatory cytokines

After injection of high doses of proinflammatory cytokines (for therapeutic reasons, e.g. TNF-alpha for tumor therapy), induction of PCT along with other proinflammatorily active proteins has been reported (238, 263). The induced levels are usually no higher than 1 to 3 ng/ml. Confusion with an infection or sepsis is improbable, since the time of injection of the cytokines is generally known.

▶ Administration of anti-lymphocyte globulins

When using anti-lymphocyte globulins, anti-CD3, or OKT-3 antibodies, occasional induction of PCT has been observed (264-268).

▶ Laboratory chemical reasons for false-positive PCT levels

In rare cases, at least theoretically, circulating HAMA antibodies (human anti-mouse antibodies) that form a complex with the antibodies in the test system could lead to false-positive PCT levels. Persistently and highly elevated PCT levels would be expected in such a case. Dilution series or the addition of mouse IgG in the laboratory could confirm or exclude this case. HAMA reactions have only been observed in semiquantitative PCT tests to date.

8.2. Induction of PCT after surgical interventions and trauma

PCT can be induced after surgery or trauma. The levels depend on the type and extent of the surgery or trauma, as well as on the individual condition. Post-traumatic induction is independent of infections or sepsis. It is probably due to tissue trauma or the subsequent systemic inflammatory response (137, 269-271). Elevated PCT levels are only found after severe tissue trauma (e.g. polytrauma), but often when patients develop SIRS or have an elevated catecholamine requirement. This has been observed, for example, after heart surgery or abdominal operations (137, 269).

The induction of PCT after operations
- is typical for operations and depends on the type and severity of the operation
- is highest after larger abdominal or retroperitoneal operations or trauma (up to more than 2 ng/ml)
- is of relatively short duration and is very close in time to the trauma (peaks on the first or at least the second day after surgery)
- does not occur in every patient
- is primarily not infection- or sepsis-specific
- can also indicate infections or sepsis
- is associated with increased general risk of postoperative complications (SIRS, reoperation, bleeding, longer intensive care stay, infections)
- can be better differentiated from septic progression with a daily comparative measurement than with a single measurement.

▶ Type and extent of surgery

After smaller surgeries or slight trauma, PCT induction is generally low or entirely absent (☞ Figures 8.1, 8.2 and Table 8.2). Levels usually remain below the limit value of 0.5 ng/ml important for the diagnosis of sepsis (21, 131, 132, 137, 272-274).

A measurable induction of PCT is more frequent after larger abdominal and retroperitoneal surgery or abdominal trauma (☞ Figures 8.1, 8.2 and Table 8.2) (128, 129, 272). Here, postoperative peak value of up to 2 ng/ml can be seen as "normal". Patients with elevated PCT levels develop postoperative complications more frequently than patients with unremarkable postoperative PCT levels (128, 129, 137, 270, 272, 275).

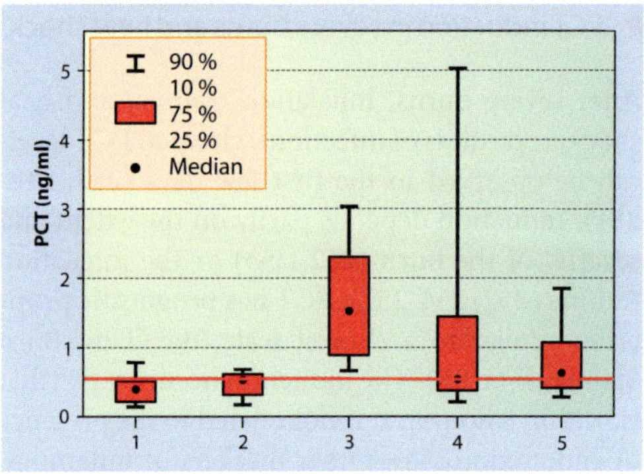

a

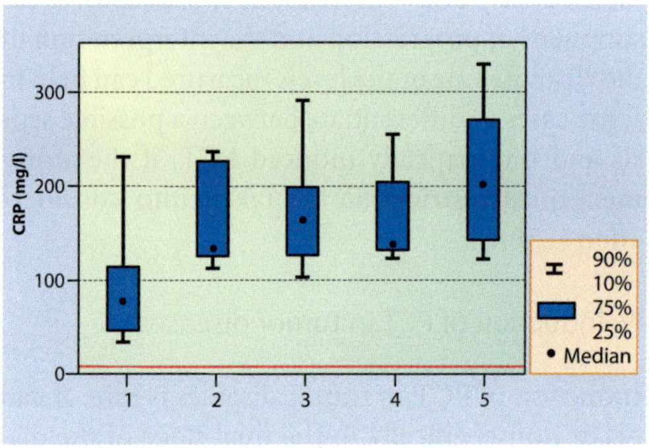

b

Figures 8.1a+b: **a:** Postoperative maximum PCT levels after different types of surgery with complication-free progression. The period of observation was up to 5 days post-op. The values shown are the median 25/75% percentile (box) and 10/90% percentile of each maximum PCT level. Group 1 (n=37) was smaller surgeries (groin hernia, total endoprosthesis of the hip, thyroidectomy, peripheral blood vessel surgery); Group 2 (n=11) was smaller abdominal surgeries (cholecystectomy); Group 3 (n=22) was larger abdominal surgeries (resections of the colon, sigma, rectum, gastrectomy); Group 4 (n=16) was extended abdominal or retroperitoneal surgeries (esophageal resection, Whippel operation, large blood vessels); Group 5 (n=23) was heart and thoracic surgery (129).
b: Diagram of the maximum observed CRP levels (mg/l) according to the types of surgery shown in Figure 8.1a (129).

Relatively sharply elevated postoperative levels are observed after liver transplantation or esophageal resection. In some cases, postoperative concentrations of more than 10 ng/ml can occur without sepsis being present (☞ Figure 5.2) (276-279).

If a patient has an increased perioperative risk or if postoperative infections can be anticipated, it is important to start a daily infection monitoring regimen with PCT early (on the first or second day postoperative).

▶ Elevated postoperative PCT levels always mean increased risk

If the induction of PCT exceeds the extent typical for an operation, various complications must be expected (39, 137, 280-282). These may include, for example, disorders of pulmonary function with prolonged ventilation, bleeding, increased transfusion or catecholamine requirement, the necessity of a re-operation, SIRS, or even infections, suture insufficiency, pneumonia, and sepsis. This has not only been determined after abdominal operations and heart surgery, but also for polytraumatized patients (21, 39, 131, 132, 137, 274, 280, 283-285).

Elevated postoperative PCT levels are always associated with a higher postoperative or posttraumatic risk.

▶ PCT in heart surgery

PCT is also induced after heart surgery. Levels are usually below 2 ng/ml (☞ Figures 4.3 and 4.4). Here, too, patients with elevated levels have complications more frequently, e.g. postoperative SIRS, increased catecholamine requirement, reoperations, respiratory insufficiency, increased transfusion requirements, longer intensive care stay, but also bacterial infections and sepsis (39, 137, 271, 284, 286, 287). This is also true of children (288-290). As early as 6 hours after surgery, at-risk patients can be detected by an unusual increase in PCT.

Daily trend measurement can also be used here to differentiate between PCT increases due to surgery and septic progression (39, 287, 291) (☞ Figures 5.9 and 5.10).

▶ What role does extracorporal circulation play?

Different studies indicate that extracorporal circulation (ECC) with normal circulation times has almost no influence on the induction of PCT. In thoracotomies, PCT levels do not change significantly when patients are operated with or without heart-lung machines, unless the bypass times are very long (130, 283, 284). The direct operative trauma seems more important, since non-invasive operating techniques also induce very little PCT. There are other previously unknown factors involved, since different cardiac surgery centers report different PCT levels (280, 283, 284, 291, 292).

▶ Induction of PCT after heart, liver, and kidney transplantation

Corresponding to the operative trauma, after organ transplants there is also a postoperative induction of PCT. After kidney transplantation, it is rather mild, after heart transplantation medium (levels of about 2 ng/ml are seen, similar to those after heart surgery), and after liver transplantation levels are sharply elevated (levels from 2 to more than 10 ng/ml). More information on this can be found in the next chapter.

▶ Induction of PCT after accidental trauma (polytrauma)

In accidental trauma (multitrauma or polytrauma) the induction of PCT also depends on the type and severity of the trauma. In isolated peripheral injuries, the induction of PCT, unlike that of CRP, is usually slight, while in abdominal trauma levels increase to ranges that can also be measured after larger abdominal surgery (☞ Table 8.2) (21, 131, 132, 272-274). Here, too, elevated levels are more frequently associated with different complications, a longer intensive care stay, more severe sepsis, septic shock, or increased mortality rate (21).

▶ Clinical consequences

In order to detect complicating or prognostically unfavorable progressions early, elevated postoperative PCT levels have also been used as an indicator for risk-adapted treatment: after colorectal surgery, a preemptive antibiotic treatment of patients with elevated PCT levels can significantly reduce postoperative infection rates (282). There are similar observations in children after heart surgery (137, 271, 289, 291).

▶ How can a non-specific postoperative induction of PCT be differentiated from induction triggered by sepsis?

The increase of PCT after an operation or trauma is short in duration. The highest levels are usually measured on the first day post-op, or more rarely on the second day. Levels slowly decrease accord-

Region of injury	Number of patients in this group		Median (10/90 percentile)	
			Injury in the region	No injury in the region
Head	67/90	PCT (ng/ml)	1.3 (<0.3-6.7)	0.9 (<0.3-5.2)
		CRP (mg/l)	115 (37-197)	121 (54-220)
Face	47/90	PCT (ng/ml)	1.0 (<0.3-7.9)	1.4 (<0.3-5.4)
		CRP (mg/l)	109 (19-206)	121 (56-193)
Thorax	72/90	PCT (ng/ml)	1.31 (<0.3-6.4)	0.75 (<0.3-5.0)
		CRP (mg/l)	115 (32-194)	136 (72-222)
Abdomen	44/90	PCT (ng/ml)	2.32 (<0.3-12)	0.67 (<0.3-5.0)
		CRP (mg/l)	136 (41-217)	107 (36-173)
Extremities	71/90	PCT (ng/ml)	1.3 (<0.3-6.5)	0.85 (<0.3-5.0)
		CRP (mg/l)	120 (48-186)	97 (11-226)
Surface	45/90	PCT (ng/ml)	1.03 (<0.3-6.0)	1.56 (<0.3-7.0)
		CRP (mg/l)	120 (43-178)	120 (14-220)

Table 8.2: Nonspecific increase in procalcitonin (PCT) and C-reactive protein (CRP) after accidental trauma (0 to 48 hour maximum of serum levels for PCT and 0 to 72 hours for CRP). The figures given are the serum levels for trauma in each region in comparison with patients with no trauma in that region. Only in abdominal trauma do levels differ significantly from other localizations of the trauma ($p<0.004$, MWU text, corresponding to an alpha error of 2.5%) (21).

ing to the half-life or slightly more slowly, and usually return to the normal range within a few days (128, 129, 272). An extrapolation of the decay rate for average PCT levels was calculated by Lindberg et al. (128).

> In contrast with CRP, PCT can also be used as a sepsis marker after larger surgeries or severe trauma.
> However, a trend measurement must be carried out in order to be able to differentiate the trauma-associated formation of PCT from a sepsis-triggered induction (daily PCT level measurement starting on the first day post-op).

Taking its general kinetics into consideration, PCT can thus also be used postoperatively as a marker of infection and sepsis: If the peak levels are documented and a daily trend measurement carried out, the expected spontaneous postoperative progression can be differentiated from developing sepsis. In that case, levels decrease more slowly, and are often higher than expected or even start to increase as time goes on (39, 40, 291).

Different studies have shown that PCT level measurement can be used even after larger operations to diagnose sepsis (for example after liver and kidney transplantation, heart surgery, lung surgery) (☞ Figure 5.2) (37, 39, 276, 291, 293).

▶ Comparison with CRP and interleukin-6

In contrast with PCT, CRP is also induced after smaller operations or mild trauma, in medium to high concentrations (☞ Table 8.2, Figure 8.2). The kinetics of induction, like the decay rate of CRP, is much slower than for PCT (☞ Figure 5.9 and Figure 5.10). It can sometimes last up to three days until the peak value is reached, and more than a week until values decrease again (☞ Figure 5.10) (128, 129, 270, 272, 276, 279, 289). The specificity of CRP for the diagnosis of postoperative infections or other postoperative risks is therefore low. In addition to this, the peak levels of CRP correlate only slightly with the severity of sepsis, and there may be suppression of cytokine and CRP synthesis due to steroids or other immune suppressants.

Unlike CRP, IL-6 levels, like those of PCT, correlate with operative trauma. IL-6 normalizes quickly after surgery (289). In some studies, the plasma level correlated with the occurrence of postoperative infections and other complications (270), while in other studies, this was not found (270). However, IL-6, like other cytokines, lacks relative infection specificity, an important prerequisite for good diagnosis of sepsis.

8.3. PCT after organ transplantation

PCT is also induced temporarily after organ transplantation. Immune suppressants administered in conjunction with transplantation clearly do not suppress this induction significantly (37, 276, 287). This is important, since it is precisely after transplantation that a bacterial sepsis must be detected quickly and differentiated from other causes of an inflammatory response (e.g. rejection reaction, viral infection, normal progression). This has clinical consequences: for infections, immune suppression may need to be reduced and antibiotic therapy increased, while for a rejection reaction more intensive immune suppression may be necessary.

In this context, it must be noted that PCT may be induced by the administration of anti-lymphocyte globulins (e.g. anti-CD3 or OKT-3 antibodies (☞ also Section 8.1.).

> The induction of PCT, in contrast to IL-6 or CRP, is not suppressed by the administration of normal immune suppressants after organ transplantation.

▶ Liver transplantation

After liver transplantation, PCT is almost always induced (☞ Figure 5.2) (276, 278). Since complications like infections and sepsis are particularly dangerous in this surgery, it is recommended that PCT levels be measured daily starting on the first day after surgery. Figure 5.2 shows the progression of PCT in patients with sepsis or an acute rejection reaction after liver transplantation.

The cause for the strong induction of PCT after liver transplantation may possibly be the increased hepatic synthesis of the previously ischemic liver (75, 277, 294), or it may be based on the increased exposition of bacterial endotoxins in the anhepatic phase, or the temporarily restricted hepatic endotoxin clearance of the transplanted liver. One possible cause may also be increased perioperative intestinal bacterial translocation due to temporarily restricted portal vein perfusion (73).

Previously unpublished cases allow us to suppose that even complete ischemia or necrosis of the liver can lead to an increase in PCT. The differential diagnosis of elevated PCT after liver transplantation must therefore always take different clinical options into consideration and evaluate them.

▶ Heart and heart-lung transplantation

The induction of PCT after heart or heart-lung transplantation does not differ significantly from the progression of other heart surgery (287). PCT levels that increase on the first or second day post-op to up to 2 ng/ml should be no cause for alarm if they decrease again quickly. PCT concentrations exceeding 10 ng/ml, however, should in any case be considered an indication of severe infection or sepsis (122, 295-297).

Even after heart transplantation, trend measurement can better differentiate septic complications from normal progression or transplant rejection than can the measurement of single values measured only after there is suspicion, as long as prolonged cardiogenic shock and high catecholamine requirement does not also induce PCT (☞ Figure 5.2). It is known that during severe cardiogenic shock PCT may be induced without a bacterial focus (☞ Section 8.1.) (233, 234, 290).

Before transplantation, PCT levels measured in the donor can provide indications of the later success of the transplantation. Similar to elevated troponin T levels, the complication rate in the recipient was found to be higher when the organ donor previously had high PCT levels (298). As a limit value, 2 ng/ml can also be assumed in this case (89% specificity, 36% sensitivity).

▶ Kidney transplantation

After kidney transplantation, only a little PCT is usually induced (37, 266, 299, 300). Since infections and sepsis are relatively rare after this surgery, routine PCT level measurement is generally not necessary. In case of suspicion of infection or sepsis, however, any elevated PCT level should be interpreted as an indication of sepsis, although post-operative induction can occur and patients with existing severe renal insufficiency and dialysis (including peritoneal dialysis) can exhibit slightly elevated basal PCT levels (☞ Section 8.4.) (301-303).

Comparison of PCT, CRP, temperature, and leukocyte counts in patients with infections, rejection reactions, or normal progression has shown that PCT or CRP can better differentiate between infection or sepsis and a rejection reaction or normal progression than can conventional and clinical markers (37). Moreover, PCT reflects the severity of a possible systemic inflammatory response better than CRP.

8.4. PCT in renal insufficiency

PCT can also be used diagnostically in patients with renal insufficiency. About a third of PCT in healthy people is eliminated renally, and patients with sharply elevated retention levels can have elevated basal levels of PCT, but there is no accumulation. With respect to peak levels, only the "plasma half-life" is somewhat extended.

If the clinically observed disappearance rates in intensive care for patients with renal insufficiency are compared with those of patients with healthy kidneys, for anuria the median plasma disappearance rate is about a third longer. The median 50% plasma disappearance rate for normal kidney function was about 30 hours (lowest quartile: 22 to 25 hours), for patients with severe kidney insufficiency (creatinine clearance under 30 ml/min) about 40 hours (depending on the study, 33 to 44 hours, with the lowest quartile at 26 to 36 hours) (27, 28).

> In kidney disease, the disappearance rate of PCT can be somewhat slowed, but there is no accumulation of PCT.

▶ Elevated basal PCT level in patients with renal insufficiency

Given mild renal insufficiency in otherwise healthy patients, PCT levels are generally not significantly elevated (PCT <0.5 ng/ml). Only at a higher severity of renal insufficiency or in dialysis patients can elevated PCT plasma levels be measured that exceed the range of 0.5 ng/ml important for sepsis diagnosis (301). Levels of more than 0.5 ng/ml to more than 1.5 ng/ml have been described, and in rare cases even higher values (304, 301, 305). Postoperatively, in patients with severe renal insufficiency (creatinine clearance under 50 ml/min) with and without infections, a shift of the normal range upwards was also observed (e.g., shift of the diagnostic limit value from 0.8 to 2.6 ng/ml for the diagnosis of infection after operations on the aorta (n=67 patients) (364).

Some authors thus recommend the use of an adjusted reference range from 0.5 to 1.5 ng/ml in patients with severe renal insufficiency (e.g. creatinine clearance under 25 ml/min) or undergoing dialysis. Since a nonspecific increase in PCT level is not general, however, even in these patients the clinical suspicion of infection or sepsis and elevated PCT levels is reason to think immediately of sepsis. If this is clinically excluded, the elevated values can be explained by the renal insufficiency or dialysis. In this manner, PCT can also be used for the diagnosis of severe infection and sepsis in patients with severe renal insufficiency, even postoperatively (303, 364).

Elevated PCT levels were found particularly often in patients with previously untreated renal insufficiency requiring dialysis before dialysis was started. Levels in this case were often 1.5 ng/ml or higher. Once dialysis cycles were started and retention rates decreased, there was a decrease of PCT levels to a range under 0.5 ng/ml; this decrease cannot be explained solely by the PCT elimination due to dialysis (305-307).

> Patients with more severe renal insufficiency can have slightly elevated basal PCT levels (frequently around 0.5 ng/ml).
> In severe, untreated renal insufficiency, higher concentrations have been observed. Some authors recommend a higher reference range of up to 1.5 ng/ml.

▶ Renal elimination and measurement of PCT in the urine

PCT level measurement in the urine is not practical, since a variety of quantities can be measured depending on the concentration of the urine. Commercial test methods are also not intended for this use. As an approximation, it can be assumed that PCT levels in the urine are about a third of the plasma concentration (28). Renal plasma PCT clearance is on the order of 0.5 ml/min. Taking physiological variation into consideration, this corresponds to a renal elimination over 12 hours of 8% to 32% of the quantity of PCT circulating in the plasma. With renal insufficiency, this value decreases to less than 3% (28). For a creatinine clearance of 31 to 95 ml/min, PCT clearance was 0.18 ml/min on average; in severe renal insufficiency (creatinine clearance under 30 ml/hr) it was less than 0.02 ml/min (28). The renal elimination of PCT is still not the deciding factor for the plasma level. In hemofiltration, significantly higher quantities of PCT are sometimes eliminated from the plasma without any permanent reduction in PCT levels (308), and in complete anuria there is also no accumulation of PCT.

▶ Hemofiltration, hemodiafiltration, dialysis

Hemofiltration or hemodiafiltration is often necessary for intensive care patients with organ failures. Since PCT is a relatively small protein, with a size just above the separation range of different dialysis membranes (molecular weight 114-116 kDaltons), different quantities of PCT can be eliminated depending on the procedure.

Studies have shown that hemofiltration and hemodiafiltration eliminate sometimes significantly quantities of PCT from the plasma (308-310). The influence on plasma levels varies, and depends on the approach taken (low- or high-flow procedures), filter membrane, and the type of elimination procedure (hemofiltration, hemodiafiltration, dialysis): some studies report a medium to strong (up to 50%) decrease in the PCT plasma level as a consequence of hemofiltration (only for high-flow), while others show no significant influence (low-flow), although significant quantities of PCT were eliminated (308-311). After changing filters, the elimination of PCT is highest in the first few hours due to adsorption on the filter (308-310).

It can be stated that even PCT levels elevated by hemofiltration are only modified in their absolute value within certain boundaries. The changes are most significant at the start of kidney replacement therapy and in the first few hours of filtration. A reduction or elimination of PCT to the normal range is generally not observed. The marker can therefore – taking the restrictions listed here into consideration – be used for the diagnosis and progression evaluation of critically ill patients even with extracorporal kidney replacement therapy procedures and for patients with kidney disease.

▶ Peritoneal dialysis and hemodialysis

In patients undergoing peritoneal dialysis or outpatient extracorporal hemodialysis, slightly elevated PCT levels in the range of 0.5 ng/ml have also been observed (301, 306). Depending on the filters used, induction of PCT can occur after hemodialysis using less biocompatible membranes, e.g. when using polyamide filters (increase by about 1 ng/ml, 4 hours after dialysis) (374). This should be taken into consideration in the diagnosis of infections and sepsis. Here, too, the use of a special reference range is recommended, for example 0.5 to at most 1.5 ng/ml, although any elevated PCT level in this range should first be interpreted as a suspicion of sepsis until that diagnosis can be clinically excluded (306).

> Patients undergoing hemodialysis and peritoneal dialysis can also have slightly elevated basal PCT levels (frequently around 0.5 ng/ml).

8.5. Tumor illnesses

Tumor diseases generally induce no PCT. Paraneoplastic formation is very rare and occurs only in C-cell carcinoma of the thyroid glands with any regularity ("medullary thyroid carcinoma"). Here, in addition to calcitonin, other calcitonin precursor proteins are produced (239). PCT can also be used as a tumor marker in this disease (239-241, 312, 366). Induction in small-cell bronchial carcinoma, on the other hand, is rare.

> Tumor diseases generally induce no PCT, with the exception of medullary or C-cell carcinoma ("MCT") of the thyroid gland.

On the other hand, in the final stages of tumor diseases, a slight induction of PCT can often be anticipated. Since levels are usually not very high, it can be assumed that this induction is nonspecific and does not originate in the tumor cells themselves.

The following data on PCT in solid tumors is available:

In 25 patients with different tumor diseases, median PCT levels were 0.2 ng/ml (range 0.1-0.5 ng/ml) (200). In another study, in 68 patients with solid tumors (57 tumors in the throat and head region) with paraneoplastic fever, levels were in the range of 0.26 ng/ml (median; range 0.05-1.17 ng/ml, n=19), and in infections the median level was 0.44 ng/ml (range 0.09-57.4 ng/ml, p=0.01, MWU test, n=35). The CRP values were the same in both groups (313). 63 adults with solid tumors and febrile neutropenia after chemotherapy had median PCT levels of 0.21 ng/ml (95% confidence interval 0.29-0.32 ng/ml, maximum level 1.43 ng/ml) (186). The following tumors were examined in this group: mammary carcinoma, small- and non-small-cell bronchial carcinoma, intraabdominal and intestinal tumors. The period since the last chemotherapy was 12 days on average (186). It should be noted in this study that the PCT level measurement was not done with highly sensitive measurement procedures, so that any value below 0.2 to 0.3 ng/ml must be estimated as a technical gray zone that may not precisely reflect the concentrations actually present.

In 23 patients with gastric carcinoma, PCT levels were found to be 0.42 ± 0.19 ng/ml (no infection). With infections, the values measured were 0.79 ± 0.27 ng/ml (314). The stage of the disease had no significance. This data is remarkable since the increase is so significant. Paraneoplastic formation or other factors may play a role in this situation. More studies should be done to confirm these results.

In patients with extensive metastasis, slightly elevated PCT levels have also been observed. Patients with liver metastases had PCT levels around 0.5 ng/ml, and with generalized metastasis up to more than 1 ng/ml (242).

8.6. Hematological/oncological illnesses, chemotherapy

For hematological/oncological diseases, no paraneoplastic formation of PCT is generally observed. However, PCT levels can be elevated in some patients with hematological tumor diseases or undergoing chemotherapy. This was observed, for example, in children with acute lymphoblastic leukemia (ALL), acute myeloid leukemia (AML), and B-cell and Hodgkin's lymphoma (244, 315, 316, 388).

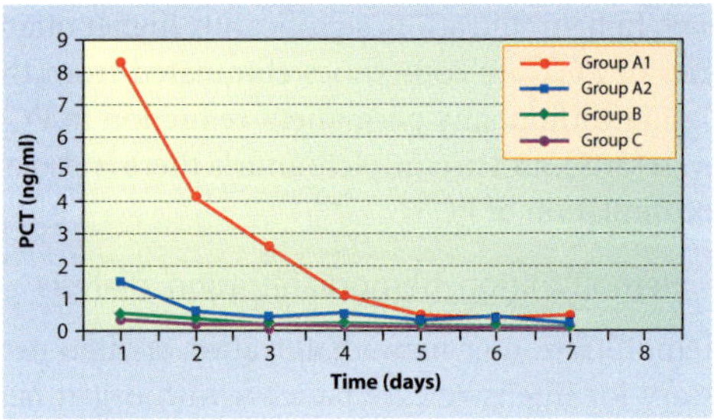

a

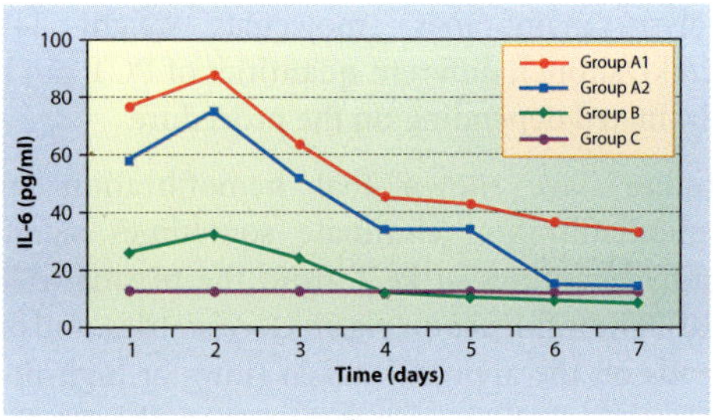

b

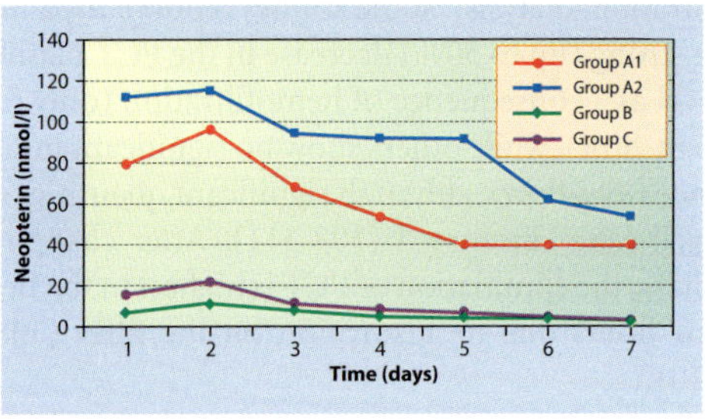

c

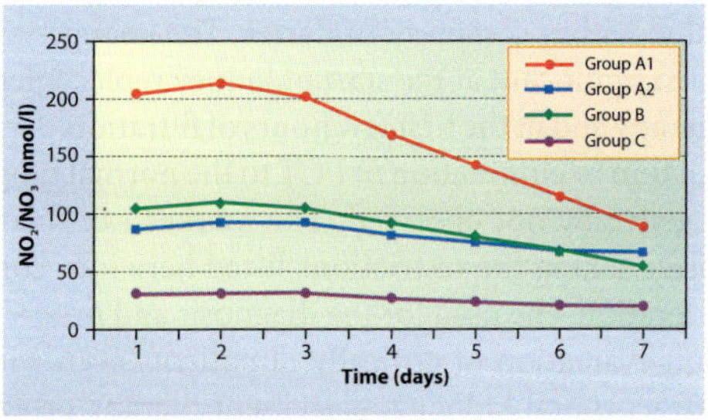

d

Figures 8.2a-d: Diagram of the serum levels of PCT **(a)**, IL-6 **(b)**, neopterin **(c)** and NO_2/NO_3 **(d)** in children with acute lymphoblastic leukemia on chemotherapy. Group A1: 18 children with fever and infection (60 episodes), group A2: 11 children with fever and viral infection or FUO, group B: 20 children with neutropenia without fever (56 episodes) and group C: 13 children without fever and without neutropenia (58 episodes with chemotherapy) (388).

The specificity of PCT for the diagnosis of sepsis is thus reduced. To achieve higher specificity, a somewhat higher limit value should be used, or one should simply tolerate the restricted specificity (e.g. using a limit value of 0.5 ng/ml to 1 ng/ml) (315, 317). At a limit value of 0.5 ng/ml, the sensitivity and specificity of PCT for the diagnosis of a gram-negative bacteremia was 60% and 85%, and for the diagnosis of a fever of unknown origin ("FUO") they were 95% and 35% (315). Other markers generally provide no better results (☞ Figures 8.2-8.4) (318).

In these diseases, too, when looking at the measured PCT levels it is important to consider whether in the appropriate studies patients with simple "bacteremia" or only microbiologically positive detection of microorganisms were studied or whether the patients had a clinically relevant "systemic inflammatory reaction" of the body as a reaction to the infection (e.g. sepsis, severe sepsis, septic shock of varying degree). The level of the induced PCT values is in individual cases also dependent on the type of infection or disease and the extent of the systemic inflammatory reaction (☞ Figures 8.2-8.4).

Clinical studies taking these relationships into consideration reach different results with respect to the induced PCT levels and associated diagnostic sensitivity and specificity. In an international multicenter study of 158 patients with neutropenia and fever, PCT levels for local infections or "fever of unknown origin (FUO)" were about 1 ng/ml, for bacteremia around 3 ng/ml, but for severe sepsis even on the first day about 14 ng/ml (average) (320).

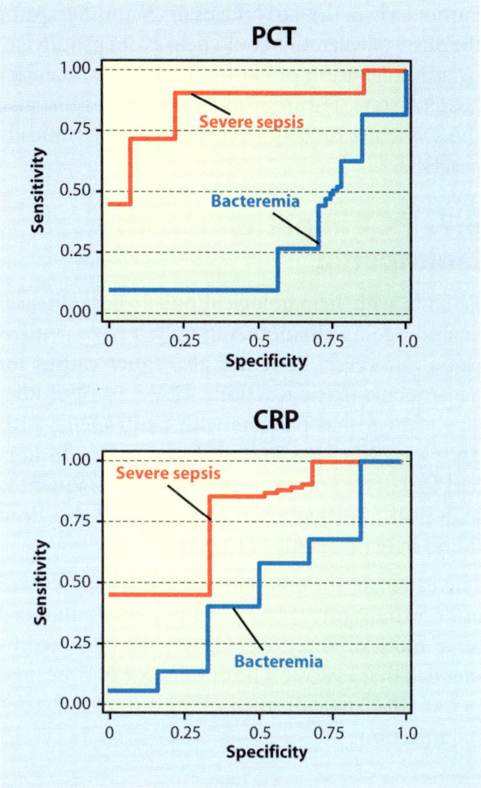

Figure 8.3: Sensitivity and specificity diagram (ROC graphs) of PCT and CRP for the diagnosis of severe sepsis and bacteremia in patients with neutropenia and fever (320). At a limit value of less than 0.5 ng/ml for PCT, the diagnosis of an infection is improbable; for values above 5 ng/ml, the diagnosis of severe sepsis is highly probable (PCT (values in parentheses for CRP, limit value 3.2 mg/l): sensitivity 83% (100%), specificity 100% (5%), positive predictive value 100% (39%), negative predictive value 91% (100%)). This data shows that the simple detection of bacteria in the blood circulation (bacteremia) need not be directly related to the severity of the disease or the PCT levels, if the reaction of the organism (the severity of the "systemic inflammation") is not taken into consideration.

PCT can also be used as a marker for infection and the severity of inflammation in hematological/oncological diseases.
As in other patients, the severity of the systemic inflammatory response plays a role.

It is presumably a good idea in these patients to use the high negative predictive value of low PCT concentrations (e.g. if PCT <0.1 ng/ml) with respect to the diagnosis of infections and exclusion of sepsis.

Particularly in the early stages of chemotherapy or the onset of fever, this could help avoid prophylactic administration of antibiotics and unnecessary hospital stays. Future studies, however, must also show whether such a procedure would be clinically practical.

8.7. PCT in patients with leukopenia

Patients with hematological/oncological diseases or undergoing chemotherapy often have neutropenia. However, there are also other causes for neutropenia (toxic reactions, HIV). Some studies have shown that patients with neutropenia produce somewhat less PCT than patients with normal leukocyte counts (321-324). Less frequently, high peak values of over 2 ng/ml have also been found in neutropenia (210, 325).

This can make the differentiation between "fever of unknown origin" (FUO) and bacterially induced fever more difficult (321-324, 326). It is recommended that a very low limit value for PCT be used (e.g. 0.1-0.25 ng/ml) when ruling out severe bacterial infection.

> In patients with neutropenia, the induction of PCT is reduced.
> Synthesis is not fully suppressed, however. Patients suffering from severe sepsis or invasive infections also induce significantly elevated PCT levels with neutropenia.
> A lower limit value (e.g. PCT <0.25 ng/ml) increases the diagnostic reliability of a diagnosis of a severe infection even in patients with neutropenia.

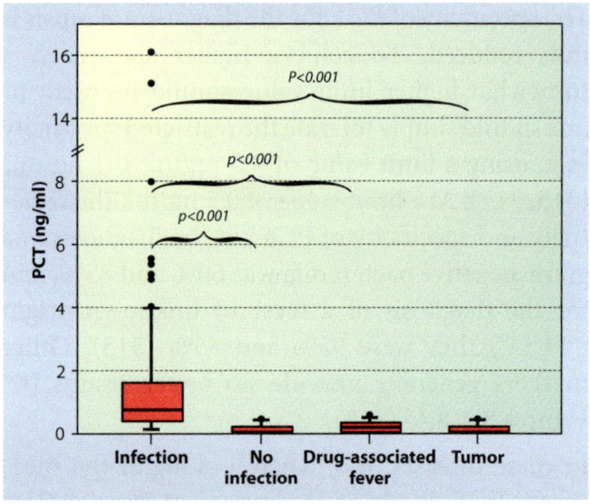

a

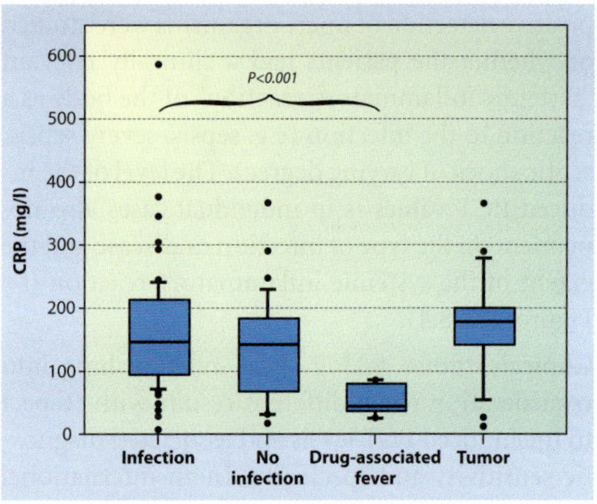

b

Figures 8.4a+b: PCT **(a)** and CRP **(b)** plasma concentrations of patients with malignant diseases (hematological diseases, such as leukemia and lymphomas, and solid tumors) and CRP increase >8 mg/l (n=111). Depicted are patients with documented infection (based on microbiology or clinical evidence), without infections (with or without fever), in drug-associated fever or patients with a heavy tumor mass or lymphomas with B symptoms (tumor group) (390).

One possible explanation for these findings could be that adherent monocytary cells, among other things, are needed for the induction of PCT. Moreover, the immune response is weakened in general in neutropenic patients. In immune suppression without neutropenia (e.g. by means of corticosteroids or cyclosporin, e.g. in the treatment of autoimmune diseases or after organ transplantation), on the other hand, the induction of PCT is apparently not detectably suppressed (☞ Sections 8.5. and 9.3.) (209).

In studies of neutropenia, the severity of systemic inflammatory response was also often not sufficiently differentiated. The symptom "fever" as the sole indication of a systemic inflammatory response is diagnostically insufficient to establish a correlation with the marker PCT, since this symptom is only slightly associated with the severity of sepsis or the prognosis of the disease. If the severity of sepsis is taken into consideration, then the sensitivity and specificity for a diagnosis of severe sepsis or septic shock were also high in neutropenic patients (318, 320, 322, 327). There is an overview study of the role of PCT in patients with fever and neutropenia for infection (Sakr et al.) (378).

In an international multicenter study, 158 patients with neutropenia and fever were examined (320). At a cut-off value of 5 ng/ml, the sensitivity and specificity for the diagnosis of severe sepsis was 83% and 100%. At concentrations under 0.5 ng/ml, severe infection was improbable. In fungal infections, PCT levels were 1.17 ± 0.44 ng/ml on the first day of diagnosis, with a quickly decreasing tendency. 12 patients died. On the first day of fever, they had PCT levels of 20.45 ± 4.48 ng/ml (average, standard deviation). Similar data has also be reported in other studies (264, 317, 329).

8.8. Bone marrow transplantation and transplantation of hematopoetic stem cells

There can also be a slight induction of PCT after bone marrow transplantation or the transplantation of hematopoetic stem cells (HSCT and SCT), just as there is under chemotherapy. The concentrations measured here are only slightly elevated (seldom higher than 0.5 to 1 ng/ml), if elevated levels are found at all. If severe infections or sepsis arise, these patients can also generate high PCT levels. For high levels of neutropenia, however, induction can be somewhat limited in this case as well (264, 316, 319, 328, 329). In these patients, future studies must show whether PCT levels, especially values under 0.1 ng/ml or observation of progression after introduction of antibiotic treatment, can be used to verify the necessity or success of antibiotic treatment (☞ Sections 2.1.5. and 6.1.).

Some example studies

Ortega et al. report PCT levels in patients with neutropenic fever of unknown origin in the range of 0.3 ± 0.2 ng/ml (average, SD), and with microbiologically documented infections in the range of 0.5 ± 0.7 ng/ml. In patients with fever persisting for longer than 5 days and a suspicion of aspergillosis, PCT levels were far higher (10.1 ± 6.7 ng/ml) (202). In 46 patients examined after bone marrow transplantation and using a limit value of 1 ng/ml, the sensitivity and specificity of PCT for the diagnosis of sepsis was 56% and 87%. The corresponding values for CRP were 100% and 41% (limit value for CRP: 50 mg/l) (319).

9. Children and newborns

9.1. Measuring PCT levels in children

PCT can also be used as a diagnostic marker for sepsis in newborns and children, as well. Working with PCT level measurement in children is essentially similar to doing so with adults (indications, interpretation of values). Numerous studies confirm this. In addition, there are diseases and indications that are primarily diagnosed in children (e.g. vesicourethral reflux, ☞ Section 7.10.). Only in newborns in the first few days after birth must special care be taken in interpretation of values: here, there is a physiological induction of PCT, but also of other inflammatory markers (☞ Section 9.2.). This limits the diagnostic sensitivity and specificity of numerous measurements of inflammation and sepsis (☞ Figures 9.1, 9.2 and 9.4) (262, 330, 331). The use of a time-adjusted reference range or the measurement of progression can help us out of this dilemma. With certain restrictions, PCT can also be used in the diagnosis of newborn sepsis or to control antibiotic therapy in newborns (332).

PCT can also be used diagnostically in infants and children. The indications are similar to those for adults.
In newborns in the first few days after birth, it must be noted that there may be physiological induction of different markers of inflammation, including PCT, so that special reference ranges may be necessary.

Since PCT levels normalize again a few days after birth, after about five days to a week after birth there is no difference in comparison to the adult reference range.

The indications for PCT level measurement in children are largely identical to those in adults:

- PCT can be used for the diagnosis of sepsis and severe bacterial infections.
- When corresponding limit values are used, PCT can help differentiate between severe or invasive infections and mild infections or less invasive infections (local infections, bacterial colonization, bagatelle infections) (high negative predictive value of normal PCT levels).
- PCT correlates with the severity of the systemic inflammatory response and provides indications of the possible progression of an infection or sepsis to severe sepsis or septic shock (danger of increasing organ dysfunction, PCT as prognostic marker).
- PCT can be used for differential diagnostics in order to differentiate between the causes of non-bacterial inflammatory diseases (such as viral infections and autoimmune diseases) and bacterial infections, once the systemic inflammatory response of the body has reached a certain severity.
- The high negative predictive value of low PCT levels can be used to evaluate the success of therapy and to control the indication of an antibiotic therapy, while taking clinical information into consideration.

Even in children, PCT can thus also provide additional useful information about the risk and progression evaluation of patients with severe bacterial infections, sepsis, or multiple organ failure, as well as those undergoing antibiotic therapy. The therapeutic success of a treatment (antibiotic therapy or focal surgery) can be evaluated using the progression of PCT. The following diseases and their PCT levels were especially examined in children:

- The diagnosis of sepsis in newborns and premature births (108, 333, 334) (☞ Sections 9.2. and 9.3., Table 9.2).
- The differentiation between simple and severe or potentially invasive bacterial infections (☞ also Section 9.3.) (22, 49, 50, 54, 368) (overview (335)).

- The probability-based differentiation between simple urinary tract infections and pyelonephritis, urosepsis, or vesicourethral reflux (☞ Section 8.9.) (50-54, 163).
- The diagnosis of acute bacterial meningitis versus viral meningitis (☞ Section 8.2.) (34, 99, 107, 192, 193, 336, 337).
- The role of PCT in epidemic meningococcal infections (381, 382).
- The differential diagnosis of viral versus bacterial causes of severe infections in different diseases (respiratory infection, gastroenteritis, meningitis) (☞ also Section 8.1.) (110-112, 198, 338, 375).

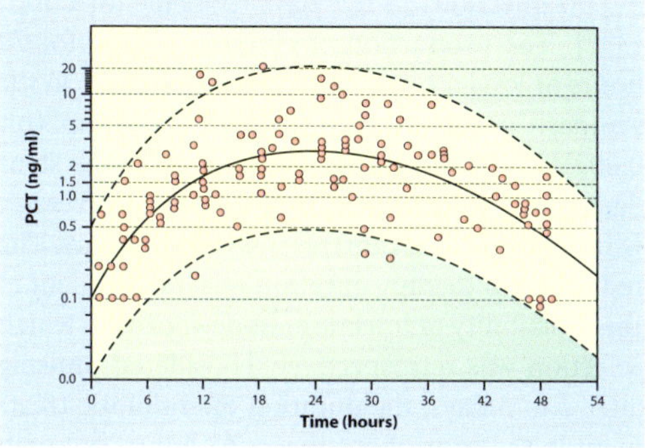

a

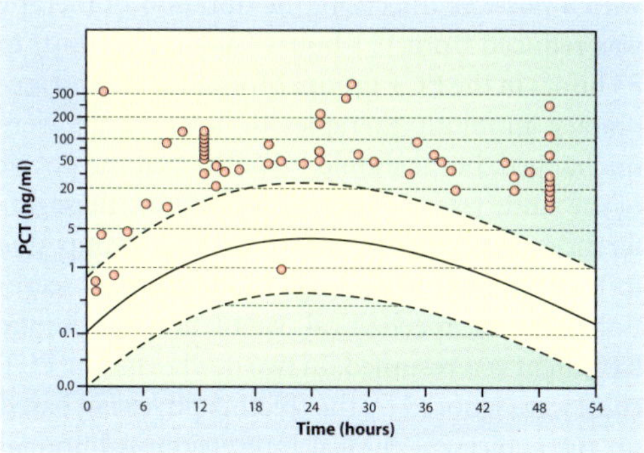

b

Figures 9.1a+b: 95% reference range of PCT in healthy newborns (n=83) **(a)** and procalcitonin levels in newborns with signs of infection **(b)** in the first 48 hours after birth. The individual measurement points are shown, with the solid line showing the geometric mean and the dotted lines the 95% reference range (260).

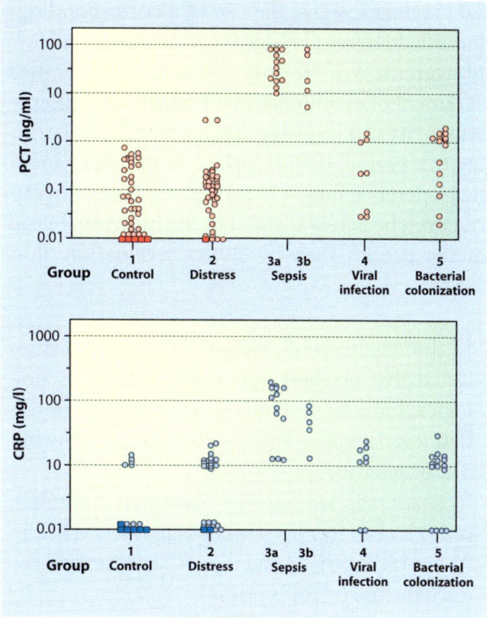

Figure 9.2: Comparison of CRP and PCT in 177 newborns. The higher sensitivity but lower specificity of CRP for systemic bacterial infections calibration is seen from the individual values (339).
Group categorization: Control group (n=86): unremarkable newborns; distress (n=50): clinically remarkable newborns without indication of infections; sepsis (n=13): clinical symptoms of sepsis and positive blood culture or cerebrospinal fluid finding (3a) or in the presence of clinical symptoms of sepsis without microorganisms being detected (3b). Viral infections (n=8): negative bacterial cultures, positive viral evidence; bacterial colonization (n=15): newborns with bacterial contamination of the integument during birth, without signs of systemic infection. For a better overall view, the baselines of the control and distress group in each case show n=10 neonates for each ■ or ■.

9.2. The first days after birth: diagnosing newborn sepsis

Newborns react to birth with a nonspecific activation of the immune system (340). This leads to the induction of a series of inflammatory markers and mediators, including PCT but also interleukin-6 and CRP. Essentially no inflammatory measurement value is excepted from this post-partum reaction. This makes the diagnosis of sepsis difficult. Unfortunately, the frequency of sepsis in newborns is highest in the first few days after birth, so that physicians are confronted with this diagnostically difficult situation. The combination of clinical diagnostic signs, the use of a correspondingly modified reference range (☞ Figures 9.1 and 9.3), measurement of the progression of values or measurement of a combination of values with different sensitivity can improve diagnostic reliability during this period. If appropriate, temporarily modified reference ranges are used, antibiotic therapy can even be better adapted to the individual needs of the patient than by clinical evaluation alone (332).

> In the diagnosis of newborn sepsis, it must be noted that newborns generally have a physiological induction of inflammation values in the first few days after birth, without necessarily indicating sepsis.
>
> If a special, temporarily modified reference range is used for this period, diagnostic reliability can be improved and it may be possible to reduce the use of antibiotics.
>
> Measurement of the progression of PCT increases diagnostic reliability. In case of doubt, the progression shows better than a signal measurement whether "normal" post-partum induction or a sepsis is involved.

Chiesa et al. and Turner et al. have created a reference range modified over time for newborns with sepsis in comparison with a non-septic control group (☞ Figures 9.1 and 9.3) (260, 330). These reference ranges, however, can only provide a rough orientation for the interpretation of PCT, since post-partum values have a relatively large range of dispersion and the extent of induction may even vary over different types of birth care and different departments or hospitals.

In a prospective randomized intervention study, a similar reference range was selected in order to use serial PCT level measurements to exclude infection in newborns more quickly, and thus shorten empirically introduced antibiotic therapy (332). Here, the following procedure was used: newborns (gestation ages above 34 weeks of pregnancy) in the first three days of life and with suspicion of infection and empirically necessary antibiotic therapy were placed in a standard group or a PCT group at random. In all the children, during the hospitalization, conventional infection parameters (blood work, CRP) and clinical progression were used independently of PCT to evaluate the probability of infection (certain or very probably infection, possible infection, probably no infection).

Only those newborns with possible infection or probably no infection were included in the PCT-controlled, patient-adapted antibiotic administration, but no children with a certain or very probable infection, which were treated routinely in both groups for 7-14 days. In all patients, an antibiotic therapy was initiated and – in the PCT group – discontinued when two successive PCT measurements were negative in the sense of the predefined age-adapted reference range (☞ Figure 9.3). In the standard group, on the other hand, these patients were treated with antibiotics routinely for three days (progression retrospectively indicated probably no infection) to five days (possible infection) (332). The proportion of children treated for 72 hours or longer could be reduced from 82% in the standard group to 55% in the PCT group ($p = 0.002$). It was shown that the patients in the standard group were treated for 102 hours on average, while in the PCT group this was only 79 hours. The reduction in therapy duration was independent of the probability of infection. In newborns in which infection was retrospectively considered unlikely after 2 to 3 days, the duration of antibiotic treatment in the control group was 67 hours, but with PCT monitoring only 46 hours, and in newborns with a possible infection, the duration of therapy was reduced from 111 hours (standard group) to 83 hours in the PCT group. Mortality rate and secondary antibiotic therapies in both groups were unchanged, but it should be noted that the power of the study was not applied to detecting these differences. In a single patient in the PCT group, due to microbiological findings in the tracheal secretions during mechanical ventilation, antibiotic treatment was resumed. In two newborns, the PCT rules were ignored by the treating physician based on the subjective clinical impression. Additional studies should therefore continue to pursue this path towards PCT-controlled therapy of newborns.

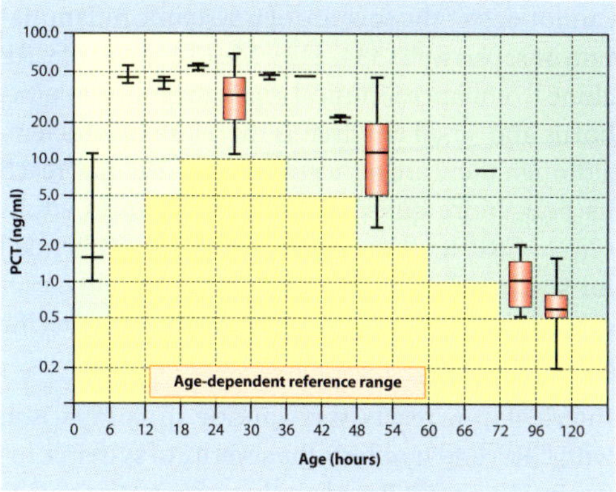

Figure 9.3: Graph of an age-dependent reference range for PCT for the treatment of newborns in the context of an individual, patient-adapted antibiotic therapy (332). The yellow area denotes age-dependent PCT concentrations which indicate a low risk of severe infection. This reference range was used in a study by Stocker et al. on newborns as an indication to discontinue a previously initiated antibiotic therapy, if there was no clinical suspicion of severe bacterial infection or sepsis but the diagnosis was still unclear or could not be excluded. The marks shown indicate the median/quartile/range of PCT concentrations of 9 patients with demonstrated or probable infections in the context of this study (332).

Essentially, just as in adults, a very low PCT level indicates the absence of newborn sepsis with high diagnostic probability, while elevated PCT levels always imply the possibility of a diagnosis of sepsis. If necessary, follow-up measurements or confirmation with other measurements of inflammation must be carried out if there is doubt about the correct diagnosis (e.g. CRP, IL-6). PCT cannot predict the development of sepsis with certainty.

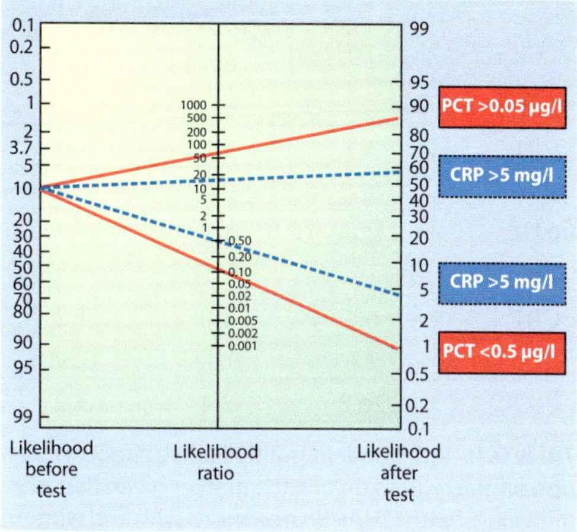

Figure 9.4: Diagram of the changing estimated risk of infection based on the test results for PCT and CRP in umbilical cord blood of neonates depending on the pre-test probability of an infection (Bayes nomogram) (386). In the population examined here, the pre-test probability (incidence) of infection was 10%. If the PCT was positive (>0.5 ng/ml), the probability of infection in these patients was 85 %. With PCT levels of <0.5 ng/ml, only 1% had an infection.

This also means that any elevated PCT level at the time of birth (e.g. in umbilical cord blood) or after the expected end of post-partum inflammatory induction (e.g. more than 72 hours post-partum) should be reason to suspect a possible septic complication (☞ Figure 9.4). This is especially important when the clinical symptoms are unclear or if measurements were carried out after the second day of life and the post-partum induced values were not measured, or do not explain this value (38, 204, 341).

Progression measurement offers the highest level of reliability in differentiating physiological post-partum elevated PCT levels from sepsis. In comparison with CRP and IL-6, the diagnostic reliability and specificity of PCT already increases within 48 hours after birth (☞ Table 9.1) (262).

	Infection	SNAP score	
		10-19	>20
At birth:			
CRP	3.7	1.2	1.0
IL-6	**12.7**	3.3	2.5
PCT	**12.5**	1.9	1.3
After 48 hours:			
CRP	6.7	1.0	1.2
IL-6	2.6	0.47	0.58
PCT	**26.2**	2.4	1.9

Table 9.1: Independent multiplicative effect of infection on the regression of each marker given (logarithmic values) with "SNAP" in newborns with and without infection (SNAP = Score for Neonatal Acute Physiology, defined in Richardson 1993) (262).

The sensitivity and specificity of different markers for the diagnosis of sepsis is limited in newborns in the first few days after birth. The interpretation of clinical signs of sepsis and the measurement of a combination of laboratory chemical values and sepsis markers is therefore essential for reliable diagnosis.
In comparison with other measurement values, procalcitonin has a high specificity for the diagnosis of newborn sepsis.

▶ Comparison with other sepsis markers frequently used in clinical practice

In the diagnosis of newborn sepsis, different inflammatorily activated measurement values are used. In addition to CRP, this includes acute-phase proteins like serum amyloid A and fibrinogen. Data on blood gas analysis and coagulation parameters can also be used to diagnose sepsis. But these measurement values also provide no complete diagnostic reliability. Markers like CRP and IL-6 are most frequently measured in many places in case of suspicion of newborn sepsis, or clinical signs are used for the diagnosis. The quick reaction time of IL-6 is generally cited as justification for its measurement, and for CRP, the relatively high sensitivity of the marker.

Comparison with these measurement values shows that each marker indeed has its particular features. CRP sometimes provides higher sensitivity than PCT. However, CRP reacts comparatively slowly and is not very specific (203, 342). CRP also cannot detect the severity of a systemic inflammation or sepsis well (334, 343). Measurement of CRP alone to enhance a clinical sepsis diagnosis in newborns and small children is therefore insufficient, although there are indications that CRP may reach its peak more quickly in children than in adults (288). CRP level measurement is recommended for suspected newborn sepsis, but it should be accompanied with at least one additional specific sepsis marker.

Interleukin-6 reacts very quickly in comparison with CRP, and it reflects the severity of systemic inflammation well. Based on these properties and its rapid reaction, IL-6 is often used as a sepsis marker in infants. However, the marker is not specific to sepsis (☞ Table 9.1). Different studies have shown that PCT is in no way diagnostically inferior to IL-6, although PCT at least theoretically has a longer induction time. The sensitivity and specificity of PCT for a diagnosis of sepsis has been shown in most studies to be similar to that of IL-6 even in an early diagnosis (e.g. when the first possible blood sample is taken after suspicion of sepsis, or when the patient is admitted to the hospital), and they were sometimes even higher for PCT (☞ Table 9.2).

Since we can only present selected publications here, we refer you to the corresponding overview works: Chiesa et al., 1998 (344); Mariscalco et al., 2003 (345); Kunz et al., 2002 (346); Leclerc et al., 2004 (347); van Rossum et al., 2004 (348); Hsiao et al., 2005 (349).

▶ Premature amniorrhexis and PCT level measurement in umbilical cord blood

In premature amniorrhexis, PCT in the mother's blood should not be the sole indicator for the possible development of sepsis. PCT may react here, but in infections in the newborn, the significant formation of PCT in the mother's blood has frequently not occurred, even if it is already elevated in the umbilical cord (350). Since these patients require particularly high sensitivity and rapid action by the physician, it is recommended to evaluate a combination of different sepsis markers in addition to conventional measurement values and clinical signs of infection, if sepsis markers are measured. These certainly include CRP, and possibly IL-6, since these markers can react more sensitively than PCT in some cases. However, it should be noted that clinical measurement values and conventional sepsis markers like CRP can significantly underestimate the severity and fulminance of a developing sepsis. PCT offers a good possibility of evaluating the progression, severity, and later the success of therapy of a developing sepsis.

In the umbilical cord blood of the newborn, PCT can also be used for the early diagnosis of sepsis. In clinical studies, PCT has a higher diagnostic sensitivity and especially a higher specificity than the comparative values examined (342). However, one must still be cognizant of the fact that the interpretation of PCT levels applies only to the time of measurement, and that the prediction of a sepsis developing later with a single PCT measurement from the umbilical cord blood is impossible (260, 262, 342).

▶ Premature births and newborns with low birth weight

PCT can also be used diagnostically in premature births and newborns with low birth weight. These children are also capable of producing PCT. The diagnostic reliability of a sepsis diagnosis was similar for PCT in some studies to that of other markers (e.g. CRP or IL-6), while in other studies PCT was better (☞ Table 9.2) (203, 262, 351, 352).

9.3. Infants (>3 days), toddlers and children

After the disappearance of peri-partum PCT induction (that is, generally starting at one week of age) PCT can be interpreted and used as a diagnostic marker similarly to its use in adults. Below, some examples of indications and studies of the use of PCT in children are presented.

> In infants (older than 3 days), toddlers, and children, the same indications for PCT level measurement apply as in adults.

▶ Diagnosis of sepsis in infants and toddlers

The symptoms of sepsis in newborns, infants, and toddlers are often different from adults. They are less specific, young patients cannot express themselves, and the illness can have a fulminant progression.

The measurement of sepsis-specific markers can therefore be most practical in these patients in order to supplement clinical symptoms and conventional measurements with additional data.

> PCT can also be used as a sepsis marker in infants and children. Despite the induction period of 3 to 6 hours theoretically required, PCT is not inferior to other measurement values.
> The specificity of the marker for a diagnosis of sepsis is generally higher than that of CRP or IL-6.

▶ Differentiating between simple infection and potentially invasive bacterial diseases

A significant advantage of PCT is that PCT can differentiate better than other measurement values between severe bacterial infection and simple infections or local infections. This is supported by the following study:

In the context of a multicenter study in Spain, PCT and CRP were measured in 445 children. The inclusion criterion was the symptom "fever" upon admission to the emergency room (49).

The diagnoses were divided into three groups based on the cause of the disease and the potential danger to the patient:

- ▶ **Group I:** viral infections
- ▶ **Group II:** usually non-invasive bacterial infections (e.g. tonsillitis or peritonsillar abscess, acute otitis media, mastoiditis, otoanthritis without osteitis, acute bacterial gastroenteritis without systemic involvement at an age above 3 months, lower urinary tract infection)
- ▶ **Group III:** potentially invasive bacterial infections (e.g. meningitis with positive cerebrospinal fluid culture, sepsis, bone or joint infections, acute pyelonephritis, lobar pneumonia, bacterial enteritis in children less than 3 months of age, or bacteremia).

The results of the study were as follows (49):

- Potentially invasive bacterial infections were detected better by PCT than by CRP (☞ Figure 9.5)
- Less invasive bacterial infections and viral infections are differentiated by both values equally poorly.

It should be noted that the differentiation of "severe" or "potentially invasive" infections in acute treatment is clinically particularly important, since an immediate calculated antibiotic or sepsis ther-

Patient characteristics	No. of pat.	PCT		CRP		IL-6		Other biomarkers		Literature
		Sensitivity/ PPV	Specificity/ NPV	Sensitivity/ PPV	Specificity/ NPV	Sensitivity/ PPV	Specificity/ NPV	Sensitivity/ PPV	Specificity/ NPV	
Newborns, including premature births, measurement on day of birth	120	87% 86% (PPV) (2.5 ng/ml)	90% 93% NPV)	68% 81% (7.5 mg/l)	80% 72%	- -	- -	Fibrinogen: 66% 80% (3.0 g/l)	91% 84%	(353)
Newborns, measurement on admission or within 12 hours after birth	76	77% (6 ng/ml) 93% (PPV)	91% 72% (NPV)	69% (2.5 mg/l) 96% (PPV)	96% 67% (NPV)	71% (10 pg/ml) 76% (PPV)	65% 60% (NPV)	- -	- -	(354)
Premature births, bacterial infections and fungal infections, measurement on day 3	35	96% (0.7 ng/ml)	84%	88% (1 mg/l)	70%	- -	- -	WBC: no difference between groups		(203)
Newborns, day 0, bacterial sepsis. Measurement on suspicion of sepsis or admission to intensive care	60	55% (7.6 ng/ml)	80%	70% (23 mg/l)	89%	55% (43.2 ng/ml)	78%	LBP: 97% (12.7 mg/l)	70%	(143)
Newborns, measurement immediate after birth	134	79% (1 ng/ml)	95%	74% (4 mg/l)	83%	73% (200 ng/l)	89%	- -	- -	(262)
As above, measurement after 24 hours	idem	95% (100 ng/ml)	96%	89% (10 mg/l)	87%	63% (30 ng/l)	71%			(262)
Newborns, diagnosis of intrauterine infection from umbilical cord blood	187	69% (1.2 ng/ml) 42% (PPV)	81% 93% (NPV)	22% (2.5 mg/l) 20% (PPV)	97% 86% (NPV)			WBC: 63% (12 G/l) 18% (PPV)	42%	(342)
Newborns (24th to 36th week), measurement upon suspicion of sepsis	200	48% (2.3 ng/ml)	97%	41% (30 mg/dl)	96%	- -	- -			(352)
Newborns (34 to 36 h old on average), n=15 with sepsis, 18 controls	33	48% (2 ng/ml)/10 %	100%/72%	48% (1 mg/l)/74%	87%/69%	- -	- -			(343)
13 newborns each with early sepsis (day 1 to 4) or late sepsis onset (day 8 to 30). .Measurement on suspicion of sepsis (day 0)	26	100% (0.34 ng/ml)	96%	81% (10 mg/l)	100%	96% (3.6 ng/ml)	90%	TNF-alpha: 100% (7.5 pg/ml)	97%	(355)

Newborns, umbilical cord blood	197	87% 98% (PPV) (0,5 ng/l)	50% 94% (PPV) (5 mg/l)	97% 67% (NPV)						[386]
Newborns >72 h, neonatal intensive care unit	176	84% 83% (PPV) (0,5 ng/l)								[387]

Table 9.2: Diagnostic reliability of different biomarkers for the diagnosis of sepsis in newborns and small children (a selection of different studies). Besides the statistical values for the time of first possible blood sample, the associated limit values for each marker, the average age and number or patients, and the literature citation of each study is listed. IL-6 = interleukin-6; CRP = C-reactive protein; WBC = leukocyte count; LBP = lipopolysaccharide binding protein.

apy is necessary, while with a diagnosis of "less invasive" or "viral infection" antibiotic treatment is less urgent and can take place on an outpatient basis or after a differential diagnosis.

▶ Other studies also highlight the role of PCT in the diagnosis of severe bacterial infections in children

In the United States, children (aged <90 days) admitted to the emergency room with fever were classified into patients with severe or presumed severe bacterial infections and patients without these (368). The following were considered severe infection (SBI): any bacteremia, any bacterial meningitis, and any bacterial pneumonia with microbiological findings, urinary tract infections with high microbial count with a dominant agent in the urine, and patients with bacterial gastroenteritis and a positive stool culture. Patients with presumed severe infections were those with a suspicion of bacterial pneumonia without microbiological findings and patients with urinary tract infections with multiple bacteria cultured. 234 children (average age 51 days) were examined. With a limit value of 0.12 ng/ml, the sensitivity for a diagnosis of "SBI" or "possible SBI" was 95%, and the negative predictive value was 96%. The corresponding PCT levels were 2.2 ± 3.9 ng/ml and 2.5 ± 4.6 ng/ml of PCT. If the patients had no "SBI", PCT levels averages 0.48 ± 1.0 ng/ml (368).

In France, 200 children with symptoms of fever of originally unknown origin were studied. 27% of the patients had severe bacterial infections (SBI) (bacteremia, pyelonephritis, lobar pneumonia, bacterial meningitis). In a multivariant analysis, only PCT, CRP, and a urine test were significantly associated with SBI. The authors formulated a score from these factors that, at a value of greater than or equal to 3 points, exhibited a sensitivity of 94% and a specificity of 81% for the presence of a severe bacterial infection as the cause of the fever (☞ Table 9.3) (380). For PCT alone with a limit value of 0.5 ng/ml, the sensitivity was also 94%, but the specificity of 68% was lower than the value of the score above (380).

PCT (ng/ml)	<0.5	≥0.5	≥2
Points	0	2	4
CRP (mg/l)	<40	40-99	≥100
Points	0	2	4
Urine test (leukocyte esterase or nitrite)	neg.		pos.
Points	0		1

Table 9.3: Score for the diagnosis of "severe bacterial infection" in children with fever (based on Galetto-Lacour (380)). For a score of 3 points or more, there is a high probability of a severe bacterial infection (score = sum of the points for the 3 parameters).

PCT is also able to detect severe bacterial infections in children with high sensitivity. An elevated PCT level in children with nonspecific clinical symptoms or symptoms of fever should therefore always be interpreted as an initial indication of severe bacterial infection.

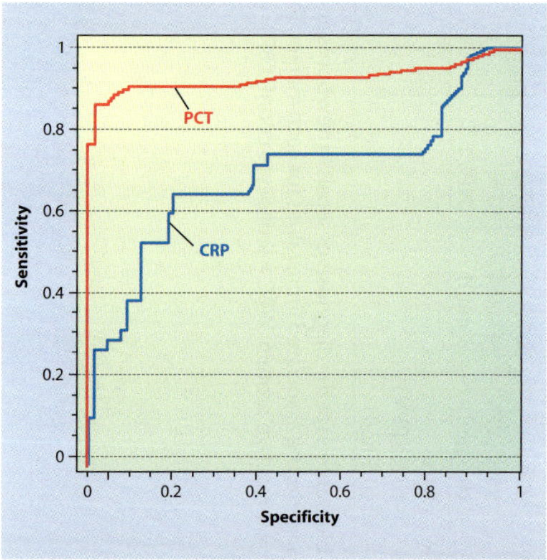

Figure 9.5: ROC analysis for PCT and CRP for the differentiation of potentially invasive infections in children with fever (<12 h). The area under the curve (AUC) for PCT was 0.93 for PCT and 0.69 for CRP (cut-off values of 0.69 ng/ml and 19 mg/l). The AUC value for leukocytes was also 0.69, with a cut-off value of 16.5 G/l (49).

▶ The role of PCT in the diagnosis of meningococcal infection

If meningococcal infection is suspected, treatment with antibiotics and possibly organ protective therapy must be started immediately. High PCT levels in meningococcal infections were associated in one study with a poor prognosis and a severe disease progression with organ function disorders. Children with an initial PCT level higher than 10 ng/ml (measured using the PCT-Q test) frequently had multiple organ failure and deaths were observed, while all children with PCT levels less than 10 ng/ml survived (382). The sensitivity and negative predictive value of PCT was 100% for the diagnosis of a MODS or mortality outcome.

Early PCT level measurement can improve diagnosis in meningococcal epidemics (381, 382).

Neither the sensitivity nor the specificity of the marker is 100%, so in case of clinical suspicion therapy must be started immediately, but an elevated PCT level need not be taken as an immediate cause for alarm, even if a cerebrospinal fluid finding is negative. In New Zealand, multiple deaths due to meningococcal infections were observed even with a negative cerebrospinal fluid finding. With PCT level measurement, 26 of 28 patients from a group of 1271 screened patients with meningococcal infection had positive test results, while only 2 patients tested negative. In another cohort of 84 patients, the sensitivity and specificity of positive PCT levels were 93% and 85%. That means that even with a negative cerebrospinal fluid finding, if the PCT test is positive, treatment should continue (381).

The PCT levels in children with meningococcal infections were on average higher than in adults. In one study, they averaged 21 ng/ml in children, but only 4.6 ng/ml in adults (381).

▶ Data recorded to date permits the following interpretation of PCT levels in children

- Low PCT levels are an indication of low risk

  A low PCT level is an indicator for a low acute-vital risk to the patient from bacterial infection at the time of examination. There is time for specific examinations, planning of additional diagnostic and therapeutic step, and any specific anti-infective therapy.

- High PCT levels are cause for alarm, also (or especially) in children

  An elevated PCT level, on the other hand, must be seen as a warning of possibly severe bacterial infection in children as well, with an increased risk of sepsis or invasive infections (335, 49, 368, 380, 381, 382). Microbiological samples taken from different possible infection sources and the initiation of antibiotic therapy should be done rapidly and without hesitation, even if no other diagnostic information is available regarding the possible cause and type of disease.

▶ Differential diagnosis of viral and bacterial infection in children

Essentially, children with viral infections also have PCT levels that are not elevated or are only slightly elevated. There is corresponding data for infections of the respiratory tract, diarrheal diseases, and viral meningitis (☞ Figures 7.2a+b) (102, 110-112, 192, 198, 338).

PCT levels need not be very high for local bacterial infections. They may even be unremarkable if activity of systemic inflammatory response is low or absent. This has been shown by comparisons of PCT and even CRP levels in patients with viral infections or local or less bacterial diseases. Here, the diagnostic clarity of both markers is not very high (49). For clinical practice, this generally is no disadvantage: in either case, antibiotic therapy would not be particularly necessary. In one retrospective analysis of children with acute airway infections, the following results were found: 132 of 327 children had negative PCT levels under 0.1 ng/ml. Of those, 38 were treated with antibiotic, 26 of those due to other causes or severe illness. In the remaining 12 patients, there was no indication of infection with bacterial agents (375).

Similar results have been obtained from studies of respiratory infections in adults (☞ Sections 7.3. and 8.10.).

If PCT levels are clearly elevated, however, immediate antibiotic treatment and sepsis therapy according to guidelines should be considered if other factors cannot explain the elevation.

Conversely, if antibiotic treatment is discontinued or not started due to low PCT levels, then various prerequisites should be noted in children as well:

- Clinical data and the suspected diagnosis should support this decision, or at least not argue against it.
- PCT should be measured with an ultrasensitive measurement procedure, since only PCT levels of less than 0.1 to 0.25 ng/ml have a high negative predictive value with reliability sufficient for the exclusion of bacterial infections requiring therapy.

- In case of doubt, antibiotic treatment should be started initially. Follow-up measurement after 6, 12, or 24 hours can then be reevaluated along with other data, and lacking evidence of sepsis or severe bacterial infection, can lead to the discontinuation of the antibiotic (332).

CRP is less suitable for the control of antibiotic therapy, although the marker is very sensitive and its measurement is very widespread. The marker lacks appropriate specificity, since CRP is also formed in viral and other diseases. Moreover, the kinetics of CRP are relatively slow, and CRP does not show the severity of the disease with sufficient precision.

▶ Diagnosis and treatment of urinary tract infections and vesicourethral reflux

Some studies have shown that PCT can provide diagnostic indications in urinary tract infections and suspected vesicourethral reflux as well (☞ Section 7.10.). In the case of more severe reflux or pyelonephritis, elevated PCT levels were observed more frequently than in simple urinary tract infections or children with no reflex disease. Here, too, the high negative predictive value of the marker at a low limit value is important for diagnosis: if the PCT level is normal in the ultrasensitive range, the probability of the presence of severe disease is low. In accordance with the specificity of the test, it was thus possible in approximately 30-50% of children with a first episode of pyelonephritis to avoid sophisticated, expensive, and for the children, unpleasant investigations because of suspected vesicoureteric reflux (cut-off 0.5ng/ml) (50, 51). An elevated PCT level may be associated with the disease, but need not be. Any elevated PCT level should therefore be interpreted as cause for alarm, since the sensitivity of the marker, particularly for reflux disease in the fourth stage, is very high (☞ Table 7.4).

10. Frequently asked questions

▶ What are the diagnostic or therapeutic consequences of PCT level measurement?

In the context of acute diagnostics or in the initial presentation of a patient suspected of sepsis or a severe infection, elevated PCT levels should cause the following diagnostic and therapeutic options to be considered:

> It should be considered whether sepsis-specific therapy procedures should be introduced, and whether the patient should be subjected immediately to intensive care.
> This includes:
> - It should be considered whether a calculated or specific antibiotic treatment should be initiated or an existing therapy modified
> - A search for the focus of infection must be carried out or intensified (including cultures)
> - It must be checked whether monitoring and optimization of perfusion is necessary in the sense of "early goal-directed therapy"
> - It must be checked whether there are organ function disorders for which therapy is required, or whether prophylactic measures must be taken to prevent them

▶ When should PCT levels be measured, and how often must the measurements be repeated?

> Acute diagnostics:
> If there is a clinical suspicion of a bacterial infection or sepsis, levels should be measured immediately.

Repetition of the measurement is recommended when the concentration is only slightly elevated (<0.5 ng/ml) and the clinical suspicion of sepsis persists. A repeat measurement is recommended after 3 to 6 hours, after 12 hours, and no later than after 24 hours after admission of the patient or the first suspicion of sepsis.

> Progression diagnostic:
> For confirmed sepsis, in patients undergoing antibiotic therapy, or for the monitoring of at-risk patients, daily progression follow-up of levels is recommended.

This is an evidence-based way in which therapeutic measures can be observed with sufficient precision in terms of their effects on the systemic inflammatory response, in order to provide indications for any needed changes to treatment.

▶ When is the use of the quick test (PCT-Q) beneficial and when should quantitative measurements be done?

Generally, the measurement of PCT using the semi-quantitative quick test is only of use in acute situations and for differential diagnoses, if no rapid quantitative measurement is available. Results should then only be interpreted qualitatively, e.g.: "PCT is not or only slighhtly elevated" (if PCT <0.5 ng/ml), "PCT is elevated" (range from 0.5 to 2 ng/ml), or "PCT is sharply elevated" (PCT >2 ng/ml). The sepsis suspicion can then be formulated in a corresponding manner. Trend measurement should only be done using the semi-quantitative test (PCT-Q) only in exceptional cases, if there are no other alternatives.

▶ Does a decrease in PCT always correlate with a good prognosis or effective therapy?

No. Of course, any elevated PCT level must decrease, particularly if very high concentrations were induced (e.g. PCT levels over 2 to over 5 ng/ml). It is normal for these levels to decrease initially. Only a decrease that persists (at least 3 days) and trends towards the normal range can be considered an indication of a good prognosis with increasing reliability. PCT levels that do not decrease consistently and remain in a range between 1 and 2 ng/ml – that is, do not quickly leave the septic range (as is possible given the known plasma half life of about 1 to 2 days) – are highly suspicious in terms of incomplete healing of sepsis and a protracted course of the disease (157).

▶ Does the absolute value of the (initial) PCT level indicate a poor prognosis or high risk of death?

No. It is true that for very high PCT levels very severe forms of disease are observed, and there is a higher mortality risk, but the course of the disease and the prognosis depend on the success of therapy in each specific case. This may be good even for a severe illness and initially high PCT level. For example, pyelonephritis or urosepsis can induce very high PCT levels. If a rapid, successful antibiotic treatment is initiated, the prognosis is generally good. This applies for other diseases as well if a rapid, effective elimination of the focus is possible. The specific PCT level thus generally indicates a high risk for the patient, but no fixed prognosis can be derived from these values (157).

▶ Can PCT be used to detect possible infections of cerebral external ventricle drainages (EVD)?

No. These are local infections that can quickly result in local damage. PCT, on the other hand, usually reacts only to a septic response. PCT level measurement is thus not sufficient for infectiological monitoring of cerebrospinal fluid drainages.

▶ Can PCT be used to exclude appendicitis or cholecystitis or an infected hip or knee prosthesis?

No. For locally restricted inflammatory reactions, even in the diseases listed above, the PCT level may remain in the normal range despite conditions requiring surgery.

▶ Can PCT be used to determine the type of a (bacterial) agent?

No. There are indications that different types of agent (including fungal infection) cause different PCT levels to be induced, but the differences are overridden by the severity of the inflammation response, so that the reliability of specificity of this differentiation in any specific case remains in the realm of speculation. The type of bacterial agent cannot be determined by PCT. No studies of this question have been conducted that have defined this question as the primary goal of the study. The value ranges reported to date overlap between the different types of agent, so that an attempt to differentiate between agents using PCT is not recommended. PCT can be used, however, to obtain indications of bacterial agents as causes of inflammatory diseases, e.g. in comparison with nonbacterial causes of inflammatory diseases like viral infections, autoimmune diseases, etc., if a systemic inflammatory response exists.

▶ Can pneumonia be diagnosed using PCT?

Usually not. However, if pneumonia is clinically probable (e.g. positive CPIS score), PCT can increase diagnostic reliability. The diagnosis of pneumonia must always be clinical. It is based on the triad: clinical symptoms with a suspicion of infection in the respiratory tract (noticeable expectoration, possibly with microbiological evidence), evidence of tissue involvement (X-ray, CT), signs of systemic inflammation (e.g. fever, leukocytosis, possibly also elevated PCT, etc.). The systemic inflammatory response may manifest in a variety of ways; elevated PCT is possible in pneumonia, but not essential: up to a third of all patients with pneumonia (even bacterial pneumonia) can have PCT levels below the 0.5 ng/ml threshold important for sepsis diagnosis – or lower. If PCT is elevated or increasing, however, one should consider pneumonia, while conversely, a normal PCT level cannot be used to exclude a diagnosis of pneumonia. In patients with respiratory infections and community-acquired pneumonia, however, PCT can be used in combination with the clinical data to obtain indications of the necessity and duration of antibiotic treatment (23).

▶ Can PCT be used to differentiate infections or infected necroses from sterile forms of pancreatitis (e.g. sterile necroses) or to obtain an indication for surgery in pancreatitis?

Only with reservations. In pancreatitis, PCT reacts to both the severity of the pancreatitis (thus to the severity of the systemic inflammatory response caused by the disease) and to possible infections. Precise differentiation is not reliable in specific cases. Both in severe pancreatitis and in infections, there is a tendency towards elevated PCT levels. The decision to perform surgery can therefore not be based on PCT levels alone. Elevated PCT levels in pancreatitis do, however, indicate a severe progression or the presence of infections with a higher probability than do low PCT levels (☞ Section 7.9.).

▶ Is there information on the basic interpretation of PCT levels?

The interpretation of PCT levels should always taken place in the clinical context. Different clinical data must therefore be involved in the evaluation of PCT. Otherwise, only rough statements on the interpretation of PCT levels can be made. As a guideline to the interpretation of PCT, the information in Chapter 2 is useful (☞ also Table 2.1 and Figures 2.4 and 2.5).

> Consideration of laboratory chemical values in the clinical context increases the precision of their interpretation.
> The diagnostic reliability of an interpretation of PCT levels is also increased when the specific details of the individual patient and the clinical condition are taken into consideration.

▶ Can PCT be elevated independently of bacterial infection?

Under different circumstances, PCT can be elevated due to non-infectious causes. A detailed list of these situations can be found in Section 8.1..

▶ Can the PCT be low despite the presence of bacterial infection?

In local bacterial infections or if, in the presence of infection, there is no or only a very weak systemic inflammatory reaction by the body to the infection, the PCT levels remain low. Local bacterial infections should thus always also be diagnosed clinically. PCT is no "screening parameter" for the detection of local bacterial infection or bacterial infection with an ineffective systemic reaction. Even if PCT is used for this, the need for antibiotic treatment should always be evaluated; in addition to the systemic effect of the infection, the local effects of an infection must always be considered (e.g. in endocarditis, osteomyelitis, local meningitis or encephalitis, e.g. if there is ventricular drainage). These and other diseases also require treatment in some circumstances even if the PCT levels are normal (☞ Chapter 6. and following).

If the PCT level is normal if sepsis is suspected clinically, it is recommended to repeat the measurement after 3 to 6 hours, and no later than after 12 hours). Since the inflammatory response in sepsis may vary in its extent, different organ systems and signs of inflammation must be considered in all cases. Besides the classic clinical signs of inflammation, there are other parameters that can suggest sepsis if there is no PCT response or it has not yet responded, e.g. coagulation parameters, antithrombin III, change in platelet counts or pro-inflammatory cytokines (e.g. IL-6). The diagnosis is thus always the result of a synopsis of all available information which has to be interpreted in the clinical context.

▶ Is an individual, patient-adapted antibiotic therapy possible using PCT and the monitoring of signs of inflammation?

Yes. Information on the "severity of the systemic inflammatory response" due to a possible infection includes a variety of information. This includes the risk to the patient of suffering damage due to a systemic inflammatory response to infection. This information, along with additional clinical information, has an influence on the decision whether an antibiotic treatment should be started or not, and on the question of whether current treatment is effective or not. The progression of the disease and thus the success of treatment must also be evaluated by monitoring signs of inflammation. This information has an influence on the possible duration of treatment and the indications for therapy with antibiotics (☞ Section 2.1.5. and Chapters 6. and following).

11. Literature

1. Morgenthaler NG, Struck J, Fischer-Schulz C, Seidel-Mueller E, Beier W, Bergmann A. Detection of procalcitonin (PCT) in healthy controls and patients with local infection by a sensitive ILMA. Clin Lab 2002;48: 263-270.

2. Vincent JL, Moreno R, Takala J, Willats S, De Medonca A, Bruining H, et al. The SOFA (Sepsis-related Organ Failure Assessment) score to describe organ dysfunction/failure. Intens Care Med 1996;22:707-710.

3. Rangel-Frausto MS, Pittet D, Costigan M, Hwang T, Davis C, Wenzel RP. The natural history of the systemic inflammatory response syndrome (SIRS). JAMA 1995; 273:117-123.

4. Vincent JL, Sakr Y, Sprung CL, Ranieri VM, Reinhart K, Gerlach H, et al. Sepsis in European intensive care units: Results of the SOAP study. Crit Care Med 2006; 34:344-354.

5. Anonymous. American College of Chest Physicians/ Society of Critical Care Medicine Consensus Conference: Definitions for sepsis and organ failure and guidelines for the use of innovative therapies in sepsis. Crit Care Med 1992;20:864-874.

6. Castelli GP, Pognani C, Meisner M, Stuani A, Bellomi D, Sgarbi L. Procalcitonin and C-reactive protein during systemic inflammatory response syndrome, sepsis and organ dysfunction. Critical Care 2004;8:R234-R240.

7. Huber W, Schweigart U, Bottermann P. Failure of PCT to indicate severe fungal infection in two immunodeficient patients. Infection 1997;25:377-378.

8. Gerard Y, Hober D, Petitjean S, Assicot M, Bohoun C, Mouton Y, et al. High serum procalcitonin level in a 4-year old liver transplant recipient with disseminated candidiasis. Infection (letter) 1995;23:310-311.

9. Beaune G, Bienvenue C, Pondarre G, Monneret J, Bienvenue J, Souillet G. Serum procalcitonin rise is only slight in two cases of disseminated aspergillosis. Infection 1998;26:168-169.

10. Charles PE, Dalle F, Aho S, Quenot JP, al. e. Serum procalcitonin measurement contribution to the early diagosis of candidemia in critically ill patients. Intensive Care Med 2006;32:1577-1583.

11. Petrikkos GL, Christofilopoulou SA, Tentolouris NK, Charvalos EA, Kosmidis CJ, DaikosG.L. Value of measuring serum procalcitonin, C-reactive protein, and mannan antigens to distinguish fungal from bacterial infections. European Journal of Clinical Microbiology and Infectious Diseases 2005;24(4):272-275.

12. Meisner M, Tschaikowsky K, Palmaers T, Schmidt J. Comparison of procalcitonin (PCT) and C-reactive protein (CRP) plasma concentrations at different SOFA scores during the course of sepsis and MODS. Critical Care 1999;3:45-55.

13. Müller B, Becker KL, Schächinger H, Rickenbacher PR, Huber PR, Zimmerli W, et al. Calcitonin precursors are reliable markers of sepsis in a medical intensive care unit. Crit Care Med 2000;28(4):977-983.

14. Dahaba AA, Hagara B, Fall A, Rehak PH, List WF, Metzler H. Procalcitonin for early prediction of survival outcome in postoperative critically ill patients with severe sepsis. British Journal of Anaesthesia 2006;doi: 10.1093/bja/ael181.

15. Tugrul S, Esen F, Celebi S, Ozcan PE, Akinci O, Cakar N, et al. Reliability of procalcitonin as a severity marker in critically ill patients with inflammatory response. Anaesth Intensive Care 2002;30:747-754.

16. Rau B, Kemppainen EA, Gumps AA, Büchler MW, Wegscheider K, Bassi C, et al. Early assessment of pancreatic infections and overall prognosis in severe acute pancreatitis by procalcitonin (PCT). Ann Surg 2007;245: 745-754.

17. Clech C, Ferriere F, Karoubi P, Fosse J, Cupa M, Hoang P, et al. Diagnostic and prognostic value of procalcitonin in patients with septic shock. Crit Care Med 2004; 32:1166-1169.

18. Brunkhorst FM, Al-Nawas B, Krummenauer F, Forycki ZF, Shaw PM. Procalcitonin, C-reactive protein and APACHE II score for risk evaluation in patients with severe pneumonia. Clin Microbiol Infect 2002;8:93-100.

19. Kylänpää-Bäck ML, Takala A, Kemppainen E, Puolakkainen P, Haapiainen R, Repo H. Procalcitonin strip test in the early detection of severe acute pancreatitis. British Journal of Surgery 2000;88:1-6.

20. Seligman R, Meisner M, Lisboa TC, Hertz FT, Filippin TB, Fachel JMG, et al. Decreases in procalcitonin and c-reactive protein are strong predictors of survival in ventilator-associated pneumonia. Crit Care 2006;10: R125.

21. Meisner M, Heide A, Schmidt J. Correlation of Procalcitonin and C-reactive protein to inflammation, complications, and outcome during the intensive care unit course of multiple-trauma patients. Crit Care 2005:nn.

22. Christ-Crain M, Jaccard-Stolz D, Bingisser R, Gencay MM, Huber PR, Tamm M, et al. Effect of procalcitonin-guided treatment on antibiotic use and outcome in lower respiratory tract infections: cluster randomised, single-blinded intervention trial. The Lancet 2004.

23. Christ-Crain M, Stolz D, Bingisser R, Müller C, Miedinger D, Huber PR, et al. Procalcitonin-guidance of antibiotic therapy in community-acquired pneumonia. Am J Respir Crit Care Med 2006;147:84-93.

24. Stolz D, Christ-Crain M, Bingisser R, Leuppi J, Miedinger D, Müller C, et al. Antibiotic treatment of exacerbations of COPD: a randomized, controlled trial comparing procalcitonin-guidance with standard therapy. Chest 2007;131:9-19.

25. Nobre V, Harbarth S, Graf JD, Rohner P, Pugin J. Use of procalcitonin to shorten antibiotic treatment duration in septic patients. Am J Respir Crit Care Med 2008; 177:498-505.

26. Meisner M, Tschaikowsky K, Schnabel S, Schmidt J, Katalinic A, Schüttler J. Procalcitonin – Influence of temperature, storage, anticoagulation and arterial or venous asservation of blood samples on procalcitonin concentrations. Eur J Clin Chem Clin Biochem 1997;35/8: 597-601.

27. Meisner M, Schmidt J, Huettner H, Tschaikowsky K. The natural elimination rate of procalcitonin in patients with normal and impaired renal function. Intensive Care Med 1999;26 (suppl.):212-216.

28. Meisner M, Lohs T, Hüttemann E, Schmidt J, Hüller M, Reinhart K. The plasma elimination rate and urinary secretion of procalcitonin in patients with normal and impaired renal function. Eur J Anaesthesiol 2001;18:79-87.

29. Assicot M, Gendrel D, Carsin H, Raymond J, Guilbaud J, Bohoun C. High serum procalcitonin concentrations in patients with sepsis and infection. Lancet 1993; 341:515-518.

30. Kumar A, Roberts D, Wood KE, Light B, Parrillo JE, Sharma S, et al. Duration of hypotension before initiation of effective antimicrobial therapy is the critical determinant of survival in human septic shock. Crit Care Med 2006;34:1589-1596.

31. Lundberg JS, Perl TM, Wiblin T, Costigan MD, Dawson J, Nettleman MD, et al. Septic shock: an analysis of outcomes for patients with onset on hospital wards versus inensive care units. Crit Care Med 1998;26:983-984.

32. Rivers E, Nguyen B, Havstad S, Ressler J, Muzzin A, Knoblich B, et al. Early goal-directed therapy in the treatment of severe sepsis and septic shock. N Engl J Med 2001;345:1368-1377.

33. Harbarth S, Holeckova K, Froidevaux C, Pittet D, Ricou B, Grau GE, et al. Diagnostic value of procalcitonin, interleukin-6 and interleukin-8 in critically ill patients admitted with suspected sepsis. Am J Respir Crit Care Med 2001;164:396-402.

34. Marc E, Menager C, Moulin F, Stos B, Chalumeau M, Guerin S, et al. Procalcitonin and viral meningitis: reducing unneccessary antibiotic treatments by routine analysis during an outbreak. Arch Pediatr 2002;9:358-364.

35. Huang DT, Weissfeld LA, Kellum JA, Yealy DM, Kong L, Martino M, et al. Risk prediction with procalcitonin and clinical rules in community-acquired pneumonia. Annals of Emergency Medicine 2008;DOI 10.1016:0-11.

36. Luyt CE, Guerin V, Combes A, Troillet JL, Ayed SB, Bernard M, et al. Procalcitonin kinetics as a prognostic marker of ventilator-associated pneumonia. Am J Respir Crit Care Med 2005;171:48-53.

37. Eberhard OK, Langefeld I, Kuse E, Brunkhorst FM, Kliem V, Schlitt HJ, et al. Procalcitonin in the early phase after renal transplantation – will it add to diagnostic accuracy? Clin Transplantation 1998;12:206-211.

38. Hatherill M, Shane MT, Turner C, Ratnavel N, Murdoch IA. Procalcitonin and cytokine levels: relationship to organ failure and mortality in pediatric septic shock. Crit Care Med 2000;28:2591-2594.

39. Adamik B, Kübler-Kielb J, Golebiowska B, Gaminan A, Kübler A. Effect of sepsis and cardiac surgery with cardiopulmonary bypass on plasma level of nitric oxide metabolites, neopterin, and procalcitonin: correlation with mortality and postoperative complications. Intensive Care Med 2000;26:1259-1267.

40. Kuse ER, Langefeld I, Jaeger K, Külpmann WR. Procalcitonin in fever of unkown origin (FUO) following liver transplantation – a parameter to differentiate acute rejection from infection. Intensive Care Med 2000; suppl.:221.

41. Simon L, Gauvin F, Amre DK, Saint-Louis P, Lacroix J. Serum procalcitonin and C-reactive protein levels as markers of bacterial infection: a systematic review and meta-analysis. Clin Infect Dis 2004;39:206-217.

42. Uzzan B, Cohen R, Nicolas P, Cucherat M, Perret GY. Procalcitonin as a diagnostic test for sepsis in critically ill adults and after surgery or trauma: A systematic review and meta-analysis. Crit Care Med 2006;34(7):1-8.

43. Tang BMP, Eslick GDS, Craig JC, McLean AS. Accuracy of procalcitonin for sepsis diagnosis in critically ill patients: systematic review and meta-analysis. Lancet Infect Dis 2007;7:210-217.

44. Briel M, Schütz P, Müller B et al. Procalcitonin-guided antibiotic use vs a standard approach for acute respiratory tract infections in primary care. Arch Intern Med 2008; 168(18): 2000-2007.

45. Ho M, Hsiung CA, Yu HT, Chi CL, Chang HJ. Changes before and after a policy to restrict antimicrobial usage in upper respiratory infection in Taiwan. Int J Antimicrob Agents 2004;23:438-445.

46. Albrich WC, Monnet DL, Harbarth S. Antibiotic selection pressure and resistance in Streptococcus pneumoniae and Streptococcus pyogenes. Emerg Infect Dis 2004;10:514-517.

47. Filippini M, Masiero G, Moschetti K. Socioeconomic determinants of regional differences in outpatient antibiotic consumption: evidence from Switzerland. Health Policy 2006;22:77-92.

48. Neupert K. Bestimmung der Konzentrationen von Procalcitonin (PCT) im ultrasensitiven Bereich bei ambulanten und frühstationären Patienten. Dissertation, Universität Jena, Germany 2009;

49. Fernandez Lopez F, CubellsC.L., Garcia Garcia JJ, Pou JF, Emergencies at SSoP. Procalcitonin in pediatric emergency departments for the early diagnosis of invasive bacterial infections in febrile infants: results of a multicenter study and utility of a rapid qualitative test for this marker. Pediatr Infect Dis J 2003;22(10):895-903.

50. Leroy S, Adamsbaum C, Marc E, Moulin F, Raymond J, Gendrel D, et al. Procalcitonin as a predictor of vesicoureteral reflux in children with a first febrile urinary tract infection. Pediatrics 2005;115(6):706-709.

51. Leroy S, Romanello C, Galetto-Lacour A, Smokin V, Korczowski B, Rodrigo C, et al. Procalcitonin to reduce the number of unneccessary cystographies in children with a urinary tract infection: a european validation study. J Pediatr 2007;150:89-95.

52. Benador N, Siegrist CA, Gendrel D, Greder C, Benador D, Assicot M, et al. Procalcitonin is a marker of severity of renal lesions in pyelonephritis. Pediatrics 1998;102:1422-1425.

53. Pecile P, Miorin E, Romanello C, Falleti E, Valent F, Giacomuzzi F, et al. Procalcitonin: a marker of severity of acute pyelonephritis among children. Pediatrics 2004; 114:249-254.

54. Smolkin V, Koren A, Raz R, Colodner R, Waheeb S, Halevy R. Procalcitonin as a marker of acute pyelonephritis in infants and children. Pediatr Nephrol 2002; 17:409-412.

55. Wrenger S, Kähne T, Bohuon C, Weglöhner W, Ansorge S, Reinhold D. Amino-terminal truncation of procalcitonin, a marker for systemic bacterial infections, by dipeptidyl peptidase IV (DP IV). FEBS letters 2000; 466:155-159.

56. Becker KL, Nylen ES, Snider R. La procalcitonine circule chez les sujets normaux. Annales Endocrinologie 1996;suppl. 1:59.

57. Snider RH, Nylen ES, Becker KL. Procalcitonin and its component peptides in systemic inflammation: immunochemical characterization. J Investig Med 1997;45: 552-560.

58. Whang KT, Steinwald PM, White JC, Nylen ES, Snider RH, Simon GL, et al. Serum calcitonin precursors in sepsis and systemic inflammation. J Clin Endocrinol Metab 1998;83:3296-3301.

59. Weglöhner W, Struck J, Fischer-Schulz C, Morgenthaler NG, Otto A, Bohuon C, et al. Isolation and characterization of serum procalcitonin from patients with sepsis. Peptides 2001;23:2099-2103.

60. De Meester I, Korom S, Van Damme J, S. S. CD26, let it cut or cut it down. Immunol Today 1999;20:367-375.

61. Russwurm S, Stonans I, Stonane E, Wiederholt M, Luber A, Zipfel PF, et al. Procalcitonin and CGRP-1 mRNA expression in various human tissues. Shock 2001; 16:109-112.

62. Meisner M. Pathophysiology and clinical use of procalcitonin. Clin Chim Acta 2002;323:17-29.

63. Nylen E, Snider R, Thompson KA, Rohatgi P, Becker KL. Pneumonitis-associated hyperprocalcitoninemia. Am J Med Sci 1996;312:12-18.

64. Le Moullec JM, Jullienne A, Chenais J, Lasmoles F, Guliana JM, Milhaud G, et al. The complete sequence of human preprocalcitonin. FEBS 1984;167:93-97.

65. Broad PM, Symes AJ, Thakker RV, Craig RK. Structure and methylation of the human calcitonin/alpha-CGRP gene. Nucleic Acids Res 1989;17:6999-7011.

66. Linscheid P, Seboek D, Schaer JD, Zulewski H, Keller U, Müller B. Expression and secretion of procalcitonin and calcitonin gene-related peptide by adherent monocytes and macrophage-activated adipocytes. Crit Care Med 2004;32:1715-1721.

67. Becker KL, Nylen ES, Cohen R, Snider RH. Calcitonin: structure, molecular biology, and actions. Principles of Bone Biology, Academic Press Inc. 1996;1:471-494.

68. Lietzmann A. Untersuchungen zum Syntheseort und zur Induktion des neuen Infektionsparameters Procalcitonin. Dissertation, FAU-Erlangen-Nürnberg 1999.

69. Monneret G, Laroche B, Bienvenu J. Procalcitonin is not produced by circulating blood cells. Infection 1999; 27:34.

70. Balog A, Ocsovszki I, Mandi Y. Flow cytometric analysis of procalcitonin expression in human monocytes and granulocytes. Immunolog y Letters 2002;84:199-203.

71. Morgenthaler NG, Struck J, Chancerelle Y, Weglöhner W, Agay D, Bohuon C, et al. Production of procalcitonin (PCT) in non-thyroidal tissue after LPS injection. Horm Metab Res 2003;35:290-295.

72. Müller B, White JC, Nylen ES, Snider RH, Becker KL, Habener JF. Ubiquitous expression of the calcitonin-I gene in multiple tissues in response to sepsis. J Clin Endocrinol Metab 2001;86:396-404.

73. Meisner M, Müller V, Khakpour Z, Toegel E, Redl H. Induction of procalcitonin and proinflammatory cytokines in an anheptic baboon endotoxin shock model. Shock 2003;19:187-190.

74. Kretzschmar M, Kruger A, Schirrmeister W. Procalcitonin following elective partial liver resection – origin from the liver? Acta Anaesthesiol Scand 2001;45: 1162-1167.

75. Kretzschmar M, Krüger A, Schirrmeister W. Hepatic ischemia-reperfusion syndrome after partial liver resection (LR): hepatic venous oxygen saturation, enzyme pattern, reduced and oxidized glutathione, procalcitonin and interleukin-6. Exp Toxic Pathol 2003;54:423-431.

76. Oberhoffer M, Stonans I, Russwurm S, Stonane E, Vogelsang H, Junker U, et al. Procalcitonin expression in human peripheral blood mononuclear cells and its modulation by lipopolysaccharides and sepsis related cytokines in vitro. J Lab Clin Med 1999;134:49-55.

77. Dandona P, Nix D, Wilson MF, Aljada A, Love J, Assicot M, et al. Procalcitonin increase after endotoxin injection in normal subjects. J Clin Endocrinol Metab 1994; 79:1605-1608.

78. Petitjean S, Mackensen A, Engelhardt R, Bohoun C. Induction de la procalcitonine circulante après administration intraveneuse d'endotoxine chez l'homme. Act Pharm Biol Clin 1994:265-268.

79. Brunkhorst FM, Heinz U, Forycki ZF. Kinetics of procalcitonin in iatrogenic sepsis. Intensive Care Med 1998;24:888-889.

80. Redl H, Schießer A, Tögel E, Assicot M, Bohuon C. Possible role of TNF on procalcitonin release in a baboon model of sepsis. Shock 2001;16(1):25-27.

81. Hohenberger P, Latz E, Kettelhack C, Rezai AH, Schumann R, Schlag PM. Pentoxifyllin attenuates the systemic inflammatory response induced during isolated limb perfusion with recombinant human tumor necrosis factor-a and melphalan. Annals of Surgical Oncology 2003;10(5):562-568.

82. Petitjean S, Assicot M. Etude de l'immunoreactivite calcitonine-like au cours des processus infectieux. Diplome d'etudes approfondies de biotechnologie, 1993; Université Paris V:1-29.

83. Meisner M. Procalcitonin: Erfahrungen mit einer neuen Messgroesse fuer bakterielle Infektionen und systemische Inflammation. J Lab Med 1999;23:263-272.

84. Meisner M, Schmidt J, Huettemann E, Lohs T, Reinhart K. The plasma elimination rate and urinary secretion of procalcitonin in patients with normal and impaired renal function. Anesthesiology 1999;91(suppl. 3A):236.

85. Wiedermann FJ, Kaneider N, Egger P, Tiefenthaler W, Wiedermann CJ, Lindner KH, et al. Migration of human monocytes in response to procalcitonin. Crit Care Med 2002;30:1112-1117.

86. Hoffmann G, Totzke G, Seibel M, Smolny M, Wiedermann FJ, Schobersberger W. In vitro modulation of inducible nitric oxide synthase gene expression and nitric oxide synthesis by procalcitonin. Crit Care Med 2001;29:112-116.

87. Hoffmann G, Czechowski M, Schloesser M, Schobersberger W. Procalcitonin amplifies inducible nitric oxide synthase gene expression and nitric oxide production in vascular smooth muscle cells. Crit Care Med 2002;30:2091-2095.

88. Whang KT, Vath SD, Nylen ES, Muller B, Qichang L, Tamarkin L, et al. Procalcitonin and proinflammatory cytokine interactions in sepsis. Shock 1999;12(4):268-273.

89. Kaneider NC, Egger P, Wiedermann FJ, Ritter M, Wöll E, Wiedermann CJ. Involvement of cyclic adenosine monophasphate-dependent protein kinase A and pertussis toxin-sensitive G proteins in the migratory response of human CD14+ mononuclear cells to katacalcin. J Bone Miner Res 2002;17:1872-1882.

90. Brucker A. Einfluss von Procalcitonin (PCT) auf die Stimulation von Zytokinen, cycloAMP und Eicosanoiden in ausgewählten ex-vivo und in-vitro Modellen. Dissertation, FAU Erlangen-Nürnberg 1999.

91. Nylen ES, Whang KT, Snider RH, Steinwald PM, White JC, Becker KL. Mortality is increased by procalcitonin and decreased by an antiserum reactive to procalcitonin in experimental sepsis. Crit Care Med 1998; 26(6): 1001-1006.

92. Steinwald PM, Whang KT, Becker KL, Snider RH, Nylen ES, White JC. Elevated calcitonin precursor levels are related to mortality in an animal model of sepsis. Crit Care 1999;3:11-16.

93. Becker KL, Nylen ES, Snider RH, Müller B, White JC. Immunoneutralisation of procalcitonin as therapy of sepsis. J Endotoxin Research 2003;9(6):367-374.

94. Martinez JM, Wagner KE, Snider RH, Nylen ES, Muller B, Sarani B, et al. Late immunoneutralization of procalcitonin arrests the progression of lethal procine sepsis. Surgical infections 2001;2(3):193.

95. Oberhoffer M, Vogelsang H, Jäger E, Reinhart K. Katacalcin and calcitonin immunoreactivity in different types of leukocytes indicates intracellular procalcitonin content. Cytokines 1998;1(1):1.

96. Russwurm S, Wiederholt M, Stonans I, Oberhoffer M, Meisner M, Reinhart K. Procalcitonin is released by human monocytes. Shock 1999;12:17.

97. Monneret G, Pachot A, Laroche B, Picollet J, Bienvenue J. Procalcitonin and calcitonin gene-related peptide decrease LPS-induced TNF production by human circulating blood cells. Cytokine 2000;12:762-764.

98. Schinkel C, Sendtner R, Zimmer S, Faist E. Functional analysis of monocyte subsets in surgical sepsis. J Trauma 1998;44(743):748.

99. Gendrel D, Raymond J, Assicot M, Moulin F, Iniguez JL, Lebon P, et al. Measurement of procalcitonin levels in children with bacterial and viral meningitis. Clinical Infectious Diseases 1997;24:1240-1242.

100. Eberhard OK, Haubitz M, Brunkhorst FM, Kliem V, Koch KM, Brunkhorst R. Usefulness of procalcitonin for differentiation between activity of systemic autoimmune disease (systemic lupus erythematosus/systemic antineutrophil cytoplasmatic antibody-associated vasculitis) and invasive bacterial infection. Arthritis Rheum 1997;40:1250-1256.

101. Hedlund J, Hansson LO. Procalcitonin and C-reactive Protein levels in community-acquired pneumonia: correlation with etiology and prognosis. Infection 2000; 28:68-73.

102. Moulin F, Raymond J, Lorrot M, Marc E, Coste J, Iniguez JL, et al. Procalcitonin in children admitted to hospital with community acquired pneumonia. Arch Dis Child 2001;84:332-336.

103. Lacour AG, Gervaix A, Zamora SA, Vadas L, Lombard PR, Dayer JM, et al. Procalcitonin, IL-6, IL-8, IL-1 receptor antagonist and C-reactive protein as identificators of serious bacterial infections in children with fever without localising signs. Eur J Pediatr 2001;160:95-100.

104. Rau B, Steinbach G, Baumgart K, Gansauge F, Grünert A, Beger HG. The clinical value of procalcitonin in the prediction of infected necrosis in acute pancreatitis. Intensive Care Med 2000;26:S159-S164.

105. Ugarte H, Silva E, Mercan D, De Mendonca A, Vincent J-L. Procalcitonin used as a marker of infection in the intensive care unit. Crit Care Med 1999;27:498-504.

106. Boutoille D, Struillou L, El Kouri D, Le Conte P, Touze MD, Potel G, et al. Meningites a examen bacteriologique direct negatif. Presse Med 2004;33:235-240.

107. Prat C, Dominguez J, Rodrigo C, al. e. Use of quantitative and semiquantitative procalcitonin measurements to indentify children with sepsis and meningitis. Eur J Clin Microbiol Infect Dis 2004;23:136-138.

108. Bugden SA, Coles C, Mills GD. The potential role of procalcitonin in the emergency department management of febrile young adults during a sustained meningococcal epidemic. Emergency Medicine Australasia 2004;16:114-119.

109. Shimetani N, Shimetani K, Mori M. Levels of three inflammation markers, C-reactive protein, serum amyloid A protein and procalcitonin, in the serum and cerebrospinal fluid of patients with meningitis. Scand J Clin Lab Invest 2001;61:567-574.

110. Prat C, Dominguez J, Rodrigo C, Gimenez M, Azuara M, Jimenez O, et al. Procalcitonin, C-reactive protein and leukocyte count in children with lower respiratory tract infection. Pediatr Infect Dis J 2003;22:963-967.

111. Toikka P, Irjala K, Juven T, Virkki R, Mertsola J, Leinonen M, et al. Serum procalcitonin, C-reactive protein and interleukin-6 for distinguishing bacterial and viral pneumonia in children. Pediatr Infect Dis J 2000; 19:598-602.

112. Resch B, Gusenleitner W, Müller W. Procalcitonin, interleukin-6, C-reactive protein and leukocyte counts in infants with bronchiolitis. The Pediatric Infectious Disease Journal 2003;22(5):476.

113. Chua AP, Lee KH. Procalcitonin in severe acute respiratory syndrome (SARS). J Infection 2004;48:303-306.

114. Gerard Y, Hober D, Assicot M, Alfandari S, Ajana F, Bourez JM, et al. Procalcitonin as a marker of bacterial sepsis in patients infected with HIV-1. Journal of Infection 1997;35:41-46.

115. Catalano-Pons C, Andre MC, Chalumeau M, Guerin S, Gendrel D. Lack of value of procalcitonin for prediction of coronary aneurysms in Kawasaki disease. The Pediatric Infectious Disease Journal 2007;26:179-180.

116. Okada Y, Minakami H, Tomomasa T, Kato M, Inoue Y, Kozawa K, et al. Serum procalcitonin concentrations in patients with Kawasaki disease. Journal of Infection 2003;48:199-205.

117. Scire CA, Cavagna L, Perotti C, Bruschi E, Caporali R, Montecucco C. Diagnostic value of procalcitonin measurement in febrile patients with systemic autoimmune diseases. Clinical and Experimental Rheumatology 2006;24:123-128.

118. Galetto-Lacour A, Zamora SA, Gervaix A. Bedside procalcitonin and C-reactive protein tests in children with fever without localizing signs of infection seen in a referral center. Pediatrics 2003;112:1054-1060.

119. Suprin K, Camus C, Gacoucin A, Le Tulzo Y, Levaoue S, Feuillu A, et al. Procalcitonin: a valuable indicator of infection in a medical ICU? Intenisve Care Med 2000;26:1232-1238.

120. Cheval C, Timsit JF, Garrouste-Orgeas M, Assicot M, De Jonghe B, Misset B. Procalcitonin (PCT) is useful in predicting the bacterial origin of an acute circulatory failure in critically ill patients. Intensive Care Med 2000; 26:S153-S158.

121. Ruokonen E, Ilkka L, Niskanen M, Takala J. Procalcitonin and neopterin as indicators of infection in critically ill patients. Acta Anaesthesiol Scand 2002;46: 398-404.

122. Hammer S, Meisner F, Fraunberger P, Meiser B, Stangl M, Hammer C, et al. Procalcitonin – Differentialdiagnose von Abstossungsreaktionen und nicht viralen Infektionen bei Transplantationspatienten. Tx Med 1999;11:54-58.

123. Zeni F, Viallon A, Assicot M, Tardy B, Vindimian M, Page Y, et al. Procalcitonin serum concentrations and severity of sepsis. Clin.Intens.Care suppl 2 1994;5:89-98.

124. Al-Nawas B, Krammer I, Shah PM. Procalcitonin in diagnosis of severe infections. Eur J Med Res 1996;1:331-333.

125. Oberhoffer M, Bögel D, Meier-Hellmann A, Vogelsang H, Reinhart K. Procalcitonin is higher in non-survivors during the clinical course of sepsis, severe sepsis and septic shock. Intensive Care Med (Abstract) 1996; 22:A245.

126. Selberg O, Hecker H, Martin M, Klos A, Bautsch W, Köhl J. Discrimination of sepsis and systemic inflammatory response syndrome by determination of circulating plasma concentrations of procalcitonin, protein complement 3a, and interleukin-6. Crit Care Med 2000; 28:2793-2798.

127. Dellinger RP, Levy MM, Carlet JM, Bion J, Parker MM, Jaeschke R, et al. Surviving Sepsis Campaingn: International guidelines for management of severe sepsis and septic shock: 2008. Intensive Care Med 2008;34:17-60.

128. Lindberg M, Hole A, Johnsen H, Asberg H, Ryding A, Myrvold HE, et al. Reference intervals for procalcitonin and C-reactive protein after major abdominal surgery. Scand J Clin Lab Invest 2002;62:189-194.

129. Meisner M, Tschaikowsky K, Hutzler A, Schick C, Schüttler J. Postoperative plasma concentrations of procalcitonin after different types of surgery. Intensive Care Med 1998;24(7):680-684.

130. Meisner M, Hutzler A, Tschaikowsky K, Harig F, von der Emde J. Postoperative plasma concentration of procalcitonin and C-reactive protein in patients undergoing cardiac and thoracic surgery with and without cardiopulmonary bypass. Cardiovascular Engineering 1998;3(3/4):174-178.

131. Wanner GA, Keel M, Steckholzer U, Beier W, Stocker R, Ertel W. Relationship between procalcitonin plasma levels and severity of injury, sepsis, organ failure, and mortality in injured patients. Crit Care Med 2000; 28:950-957.

132. Hensler T, Sauerland S, Lefering R, Nagelschmidt M, Bouillon B, Andermahr J, et al. The clinical value of procalcitonin and neopterin in predicting sepsis and organ failure after major trauma. Shock 2003;20(5):420-426.

133. Haverkate F, Thompson SG, Pyke SD, Gallimore JR, Pepys MB. Production of C-reactive protein and risk of coronary events in stable and unstable angina. European concerted action on thrombosis and disabilities angina pectoris study group. Lancet 1997;349:462-466.

134. Brunkhorst FM, Wegscheider K, Forycki ZF, Brunkhorst R. Procalcitonin for early diagnosis and differentiation of SIRS, sepsis, severe sepsis, and septic shock. Intensive Care Med 2000;26(suppl.):S148-S152.

135. Giamarellos-Bourboulis EJ, Mega A, Grecka P, Scarpa N, Koratzanis G, Thomopoulos G, et al. Procalcitonin: a marker to clearly differentiate systemic inflammatory response syndrome and sepsis in the critically ill patient? Intensive Care Med 2002;28:1351-1356.

136. De Talance N, Burlet C, Claudel C. La procalcitonine (PCT) est-elle le marqueur specifique du choc septique? Immunoanalyse et Biologie specialisee 2003;18: 120-122.

137. Meisner M, Rauschmayer C, Schmidt J, Feyrer R, Cesnevar R, Bredle D, et al. Early increase of procalcitonin after cardiovascular surgery in patients with non-infectious and infectious postoperative complications. Intensive Care Med 2002;28:1094-1102.

138. Oda S, Hirasawa H, Shiga H, Nakanishi K, Matsuda K, Nakamua M. Sequential measurement of IL-6 blood levels in patients with systemic inflammatory response syndrome (SIRS/sepsis). Cytokine 2005;29:169-175.

139. Reinhart K, Wiegand-Lohnert C, Grimminger F, Kaul M, Withington S, Treacher D, et al. Assessment of the safety and efficacy of the monoclonal anti-tumor necrosis factor antibody-fragment, MAK 195F, in patients with sepsis and septic shock: a multicenter, randomized, placebo-controlled, dose-ranging study. Crit Care Med 1996;24:733-742.

140. Marshall JC, Walker PM, Foster DM, Harris D, Ribeiro M, Paice J, et al. Measurement of endotoxin activity in critically ill patients using whole blood neutrophil dependent chemiluminescence. Critical Care 2002; 6(4): 342-348.

141. Gibot S, Cravoisy A, Kolopp-Sarda MN, Bene MC, Faure G, Bollaert PE, et al. Time-course of sTREM (soluble triggering receptor expressed on myeloid cells)-1, procalcitonin, and C-reactive protein plasma concentrations during sepsis. Crit Care Med 2005;33:792-796.

142. Siassi M, Riese J, Steffensen R, Meisner M, Thiel S, Hohenberger W, et al. k and procalcitonin measurement for prediction of postoperative infection. Critical Care 2005;9:R483-F489.

143. Pavcnik-Arnol M, Hojker S, Derganc M. Lipoprotein-binding protein in critically ill neonates and children with suspected infection: comparison with procalcitonin, interleukin-6 and C-reactive protein. Intensive Care Med 2004;30:1454-1460.

144. Marshall JC, Foster D, Vincent JL, Cook DJ, Cohen J, Dellinger RP, et al. Diagnostic and prognostic implications of endotoxinemia in criticall illness: Results of the MEDIC study. The Journal of Infectious Disease 2004; 190:527-534.

145. Kofoed K, Andersen O, Kronborg G, Tvede M, Petersen J, Eugen-Olsen J, et al. Use of plasma C-reactive protein, procalcitonin, neutrophils, macrophage migration inhibitory factor, soluble urokinase-type plasminogen activator receptor, and soluble triggering receptor expressed on myeloid cells-1 in combination to diagnose infections: a prospective study. Critical Care 2007;11: R38.

146. Stolz D, Christ-Crain M, Morgenthaler NG, Leuppi J, Miedinger D, Bingisser R, et al. Copeptin, C-Reactive Protein, and Procalcitonin as Prognostic Biomarkers in Acute Exacerbation of COPD. Chest 2007;131:1058-1067.

147. Dhainaut JF, Shorr AF, Marcias WL, Kollef MJ, Levi M, Reinhart K, et al. Dynamic evolution of coagulopathy in the first day of severe sepsis: relationship with mortality and organ failure. Crit Care Med 2005;33(2):341-348.

148. Morgenthaler NG, Struck J, Christ-Crain M, Bergmann A, Müller B. Pro-atrial natriuretic peptide is a prognostic marker in sepsis, similar to the APACHE II score: an observational study. Critical Care 2005;9:R37-R45.

149. Seligman R, Morgenthaler C, Meisner M. Copeptin. 2008.

150. Meyer E, Schwab F, Schroeren-Boersch B, Rüden H, Gastmeier P. Diversität des Antibiotikaverbrauchs auf Intensivstationen in Deutschland. Dtsch Med Wochenschr 2008;133:235-240.

151. El Mousaoui R, de Borgie CAJ, van den Broek P, Hustinx WN, Bresser P, van den Berk GEL, et al. Effectiveness of discontinuing antibiotic treatment after three days versus eight days in mild to moderate-severe community acquired pneumonia: randomised, double blind study. British Medical Journal 2006;332(1335-1343).

152. Singh N, Rogers P, Atwood CW, Wagener MM, Victor LY. Short,course empiric antibiotic therapy for patients with pulmonary infiltrates in the intensive care unit. Am J Respir Crit Care Med 2000;162:505-511.

153. Kollef MH, Morrow LE, Niederman MS, Leeper KY, al. e. Clinical characteristics and treatment patterns among patients with ventilator-associated pneumonia. Chest 2006;129:1210-1218.

154. Micek ST, Ward S, Fraser VJ, Kollef MH. A randomized controlled trial of an antibiotic discontinuation policy for clinically suspected ventilator-associated pneumonia. Chest 2004;12:1600-1602.

155. Gramm HJ, Dollinger P, Beier W. Procalcitonin – ein neuer Marker der inflammatorischen Wirtsantwort. Longitudinalstudien bei Patienten mit Sepsis und Peritonitis. Chir.Gastroenterol.suppl.2 1995;11:51-54.

156. von Lilienfeld-Toal M, Schneider A, Orlopp K, Hahn-Ast C, Glasmacher A, Stüber F. Change of procalcitonin predicts clinical outcome of febrile episodes in patients with hematological malignancies. Support Care Cancer 2006;DOI 10.1007/s00520-006-0081-2.

157. Jensen JU, Heslet L, ensen TH, Espersen K, Steffensen P, Tvede M. Procalcitonin increase in early identification of critically ill patients at high risk of mortality. Crit Care Med 2006;34:2596-2602.

158. Chastre J, Wolff M, Fagon JY, Chevret S, Thomas F, Wermert D, et al. Comparison of 8 vs 15 days of antibiotic therapy for ventilator-associated pneumonia in adults: a randomized trial. JAMA 2003;290:2588-2598.

159. Chun C, Yao W, Chen Y, Liu Z, Zhang XW. Value of serum procalcitonin in diagnosing bacterial lower respiratory tract infections in people with exacerbation of chronic obstructrive pulmonary disease. Journal of Peking University (Health Sciences) 2006;38(4):389-392.

160. Grossmann RF, Fein A. Evidence-based assessment of diagnostic tests for ventilator-associated pneumonia. Executive Summary. Chest 2000;117(suppl.2):177S-181S.

161. Nyamande K, Lalloo UG. Serum procalcitonin distinguishes CAP due to bacteriae, mycobacterium tuberculosis and PJP. Int J Tuberc Lung Dis 2006;10:510-515.

162. Don M, Valent F, Korppi M, Falleti E, De Candia A, Fasoli L, et al. Efficiacy of serum procalcitonin in evaluating severity of community-acquired pneumonia in childhood. Scandinavian Journal of Infectious Diseases 2007;39:129-137.

163. Prat C, Dominguez J, Rodrigo C, Gimenez M, Azuara M, Jimenez O, et al. Elevated serum procalcitonin values correlate with renal scarring in children with urinary tract infection. Pediatr Infect Dis J 2003;22: 438-442.

164. Korppi M, Remes S, Heiskanen-Kosma T. Serum procalcitonin concentrations in bacterial pneumonia in children: a negative result in primary healthcare settings. Pediatric Pulmonology 2003;35:56-61.

165. Korppi M, Remes S. Serum procalcitonin in pneumococcal pneumonia in children. Eur Resipr J 2001; 17:623-627.

166. Jereb M, Kotar T. Usefulness of procalcitonin to differentiate typical from atypical community-acquired pneumonia. Wien Klin Wochenschr 2006;118:170-174.

167. Schleicher GK, Herbert V, Brink A, Martin S, Maraj R, Galpin JS, et al. Procalcitonin and C-reactive protein

levels in HIV-positive subjects with tuberculosis and pneumonia. Eur Respir J 2005;25:688-692.

168. Polzin A, Pletz M, Erbes R, Raffenberger M, Mauch H, Wagner S, et al. Procalcitonin as a diagnostic tool in lower respiratory tract infections and tuberculosis. Eur Respir J 2003;21:939-943.

169. Baylan O, Balkan A, Inal A, Kisa O, Albay A, Doganci L, et al. The predictive value of serum procalcitonin levels in adult patients with active pulmonary tuberculosis. Jpn J Infect Dis 2006;59:164-167.

170. Kandemir O, Uluba B, Polat G, Sezer C, Camdeviren H, Kaya A. Elevation of procalcitonin level in patients with pulmonary tuberculosis and in medical staff with close patient contact. Archives of Medical Research 2003;34:311-314.

171. Cakir E, Deniz O, Ozcan O, Tozkoparan E, Yaman H, Akgul EO, et al. Pleural fluid and serum procalcitonin as diagnostic tools in tuberculosis pleurisy. Clinical Biochemistry 2004;38:234-238.

172. Gramm HJ, Beier W, Zimmermann J, Oedra N, Hannemann L, Boese-Landgraf J. Procalcitonin (ProCT) – A biological marker of the inflammatory response with prognostic properties. Clin.Intens.Care suppl.2 1995;6:71.

173. Michelow IC, Olsen K, Lozano J, Rollins NK, Duffy LB, Ziegler.T., et al. Epidemiology and clinical characterisitics of community-acquired pneumonia in hospitalized children. Pediatrics 2004;113(4):701-707.

174. Boussekey N, Leroy O, Alfandari S, Devos P, Georges H, Guery B. Procalcitonin kinetics in the prognosis of severe community-acquired pneumonia. Intensive Care Med 2006;32:469-472.

175. Brunkhorst FM, Forycki ZF, Wagner J. Discrimination of infectious and non-infectious etiologies of the adult respiratory distress syndrome (ARDS) with procalcitonin immunoreactivity. Clin Intens Care 1995;6:3.

176. Laupland KB, Leed H, Gregson DB, Manns BJ. Cost of intensive care unit-acquired bloodstream infections. Journal of Hospital Infection 2006;63:124-132.

177. Chan YL, Tseng CP, Tsay PK, Chang SS, Chiu TF, Chen JC. Procalcitonin as a marker of bacterial infection in the emergency department: an observational study. Critical Care 2004;8(1):R12-R20.

178. Bell K, Wattie M, Byth K, Silvestrini R, Clark P, Stachowski E, et al. Procalcitonin: a marker of bacteraemia and SIRS. Anaest Intensive Care 2003;31:629-636.

179. Peters RPH, Twisk WR, van Agtmael MA, Groeneveld ABJ. The role of procalcitonin in a decision tree for prediction of bloodstream infection in febrile patients. Clin Microbiol Infect 2006;12:1207-1213.

180. Caterino JM, Scheatzle MD, Forbes ML, D'Antonio JA. Bacteremic elder emergency department patients: procalcitonin and white count. Acad Emerg Med 2004; 11(4):393-396.

181. Liaudat S, Dayer E, Praz G, Bille J, Troillet N. Usefulness of procalcitonin serum level for the diagnosis of bacteremia. Eur J Clin Microbiol Infect Dis 2001;20:524-527.

182. Chirouze C, Schuhmacher H, Rabaud C, Gil H, Khayat N, Estavoyer JM, et al. Low serum procalcitonin level accurately predicts the absence of bacteremia in adult patient with acute fever. Clin Infect Dis 2002; 35:156-161.

183. Rintala EM, Aittoniemi J, Laine S, Nevalainen TJ, Nikoskelainen J. Early identification of bacteremia by biochemical markers of systemic inflammation. Scand J Clin Lab Invest 2001;61:523-530.

184. Engel A, Mack E, Kern P, Kern WV. An analysis of interleukin-8, interleukin-6 and C-reactive protein serum concentrations to predict fever, gram-negative bacteremia and complicated infection in neutropenic cancer patients. Infection 1998;26(4):213-221.

185. Persson L, Engervall P, Magnuson A, Vikerfors T, Söderquist B, Hansson LO, et al. Use of inflammatory markers for early detection of bacteremia in patients with febrile neutropenia. Scand J Infect Dis 2004;36:365-371.

186. Jimeno A, Garcia-Valasco A, Del Val O, Gonzalez-Billalabeitia E, Hernando S, Hernandez R, et al. Assessment of procalcitonin as a diagnostic and prognostic marker in patient with solid tumors and febrile neutropenia. American Cancer Society 2004;100:2462-2469.

187. Gras-le-Guen C, Delmas C, Launay E, Caillon J, Loubersac V, Pichoret G, et al. Contribution of procalcitonin to occult bacteremia detetion in children. Scandinavian Journal of Infectious Diseases 2007;39: 157-159.

188. Mueller C, Christ-Crain M, Müller B. What Cardiologist do need to know about procalcitonin. Clin Lab 2005;51:1-4.

189. Hryniewiecki T, Sitkiewicz D, Rawczynska-Englert I. Role of procalcitonin in diagnosis of uncomplicated infective endocarditis (article in polish). Przeglad Lakarnski 2002;59:793-795.

190. Mueller C, Huber P, Laifer G, Müller B, Perruchoud AP. Procalcitonin and the early diagnosis of infective endocarditis. Circulation 2004;109:1707-1710.

191. Kocazeybek B, Kücükoglu S, Öner YA. Procalcitonin and C-reactive protein in infective endocarditis: correlation with etiology and prognosis. Chemotherapy 2003;49:76-84.

192. Dubos F, Moulin F, Gajdos V, De Suremain N, Biscardi S, Lebon P, et al. Serum procalcitonin and other

biologic markers to distinguish between bacterial an aseptic meningitis. J Pediatr 2006;149:72-76.

193. Schwarz S, Bertram M, Schwab S, Andrassy K, Hacke W. Serum procalcitonin levels in bacterial and abacterial meningitis. Crit Care Med 2000;28(6):1828-1832.

194. Ray P, Badarou-Acossi G, Viallon A, Boutoille D, Arthaud M, Trystam D, et al. Accuracy of cerebrospinal fluid results to differentiate bacterial from non bacterial meningitis in case of negative gram-strained smear. American Journal of Emergency Medicine 2007;25:179-184.

195. Martinez R, Gaul C, Buchfelder M, Ergbuth F, Tschaikowksy K. Serum procalcitonin monitoring for differential diagnosis of meningitis and ventriculitis in adult intensive care patients. Intensive Care Med 2002; 28:399-405.

196. Jereb M, Muzlovic I, Hojker S, Strele F. Predictive value of serum and cerebrospinal fluid procalcitonin levels for the diagnosis of bacterial meningitis. Infection 2001;29:209-212.

197. Lorrot M, Moulin F, Coste J, Ravilly S, Guerin S, Lebon P, et al. Procalcitonin aux urgences pediatriques. La Presse Medicale 2000;29(3):128-134.

198. Matesanz JL, Fernandez E, Fernandez JM, Viejo G. Plasma procalcitonin and C-reactive protein concentrations in pediatric patient with Epstein-Barr virus infection. Clinical Chemistry 2003;49(12):2103-2104.

199. Lotric-Furlan S, Rojko T, Strle F. Concentration of procalcitonin and C-reactive protein in patients with human granulocytic anaplasmosis and the initial phase of tick-borne encephalitis. Ann NY Acad Sci 2005;1063: 439-441.

200. Delevaux I, Andre M, Colombier M, Albuisson E, Meylheuc F, Begue RJ, et al. Can procalcitonin measurement help in differentiating between bacterial infection and other kinds of inflammatory process ? Ann Rheum Dis 2003;62:337-340.

201. Elefsiniotis IS, Petrocheilou A, Scarmeas N et al. Serum procalcitonin levels in chronic hepatitis C patients under pegylated interferon-alpha plus ribavirin treatment. Eur J Gastroenterol Hepatol 2006;37:329-331.

202. Ortega M, Rovira M, Filella X, Almela M, de la Bellacasa JP, Carreras E, et al. Prospective evaluation of procalcitonin in adults with febrile neutropenia after haematopoetic stem cell transplantation. Brit J Hematology 2004;126:372-378.

203. Distefano G, Curreri R, Betta P, Romeo MG, Amato M. Procalcitonin serum levels in perinatal bacterial and fungal infection of preterm infants. Acta Paediatr 2004; 93:216-219.

204. Han YY, Doughty LA, Kofos D, Sasser H, Carcillo JA. Procalcitonin is persistenly increased among children with poor outcome from bacterial sepsis. Pediatr Crit Care Med 2003;4:21-25.

205. Christofilopoulou S, Charvalos E, Petrikkos G. Could procalcitonin be a predictive biological marker in systemic fungal infections ? European Journal of Internal Medicine 2002;13:493-495.

206. Jemli B, Aouni Z, Lebben I, Mazigh C, Ferjani M, Machgoul M, et al. Procalcitonine et candidoses invasives en milieu de reanimation. Ann Biol Clin 2007; 65:169-173.

207. Schwenger V, Sis J, Breitbart A, Andrassy K. CRP levels in autoimmune disease can be specified by measurement of procalcitonin. Infection 1998;26:274-276.

208. Moosig F, Csernok E, Reinhold-Keller E, Schmitt W, Gross WL. Elevated procalcitonin levels in active Wegeners granulomatosis. J Rheumatol 1998;25:1531-1533.

209. Rinaldi S, Adembri C, Grechi S, De Gaudio R. Low-dose hydrocortisone during severe sepsis: Effects on microalbuminuria. 2006;Crit Care Med(34):2334-2339.

210. Al-Nawas B, Shah PM. Procalcitonin in patients with and without immunosuppression and sepsis. Infection 1996;24:434-436.

211. Kadar J, Petrovicz E. Adult-onset Still´s disease. Best Practice and Research Clinical Rheumatology 2004; 18(5):663-676.

212. Scire CA, Caporali R, Perotti C, Montecucco C. Il dosaggio della procalcitonina plasmatica in reumatologia (Plasma concentration in rheumatic diseases). Reumatismo 2003;55(2):113-118.

213. Stroehmann A, Kuenzel K, Hiepe F, Beier W, Burmester GR, Krause A. Procalcitonin: a marker for bacterial infection in patients with rheumatic diseases? Abstract on Congress Orlando 1997;1:1.

214. Wu J, Zhou T, Zhand J, He J, Gause WC, Mountz JD. Correction of autoimmune disease by early replacement of mutated lpr gene with the normal Fas apoptosis gene in the T cells of transgenic MRL-lpr/lpr mice. Proc Natl Acad Sci 1994;91:2344-2348.

215. Purkayastha S, Chow A, Athanasiou T, Cambaroudis A, Panesar S, Kinross J, et al. Does serum procalcitonin have a role in evaluating the severity of acute pancreatitis? A question revisited. World J Surg 2006;30: 1713-1721.

216. Ranson HHC, Rifkind KM, Roses DF, al. e. Prognostic signs and the role of operative management in acute pancreatitis. Surg Gynecol Obstet 1974;139:69-81.

217. Ranson JHC. Etiological and prognostic factors in human acute pancreatitis: A review. Am J Gastroenterol 1982;77:633-638.

218. Bradley ELI. A clinically based classification system for acute pancreatitis. Summary of the International Symposium on Acute Pancreatitis, Atlanta, Ga, September 11 through 13, 1992. Arch Surg 1993;128:586-590.

219. Kylänpää-Bäck ML, Takala A, Kamppainen EA, Puolakkainen PA, Leppäniemi AK, Karonen SL, et al. Procalcitonin, soluble interleukin-2 receptor, and soluble E-selectin in predicting the severity of acute pancreatitis. Crit Care Med 2001;29:63-69.

220. Bülbüller N, Dogru O, Ayten R, Akbulut H, Ilhan YS, Cetinkaya Z. Procalcitonin is a predictive marker for severe acute pancreatitis. Turkish Journal of Trauma and Emergency Surgery 2006;12(2):115-120.

221. Mandi Y, Farkas G, Takacs T, Boda K, Lonovics J. Diagnostic relevance of procalcitonin, IL-6,and sICAM-1 in the prediction of infected necrosis in acute pancreatitis. Int I Pancreatol 2000;28:41-49.

222. Yonetci N, Sungurtekin U, Oruc N, Yilmaz M, Sungurtekin H, Kaleli I, et al. Is procalcitonin a reliable marker for the diagnosis of infected pancreatic necrosis? ANZ J Surg 2004;74:591-595.

223. Olah A, Belagyi T, Issekutz A, Makay R, Zaborszky A. Differentiation between sterile and infected forms of acute pancreatitis. Hepato-Gastroenterology 2005;52: 243-245.

224. Bertsch T, Richter A, Hofheinz H, Bohm C, Hartel M, Aufenanger J. Procalcitonin. A new marker for acute phase reaction in acute pancreatitis. Langenbecks Arch Chir 1997;382:367-372.

225. Müller CA, Uhl W, Printzen G, Gloor B, Bischofberger H, Tcholakov O, et al. Role of procalcitonin and granulocyte colony stimulating factor in the early prediction of infected necrosis in severe acute pancreatitis. Gut 2000;46:233-238.

226. Makay R, Issekuz A. Procalcitonin gyorsteszt szerepe az akut necrotizalo pancreatitis steril es inficalt formaink e. Magyar Sebeszet 2003;56:31-33.

227. Riche FC, Cholley BP, Laisne MJC, Vicaut E, Panis YH, Lajeunie EJ, et al. Inflammatory cytokines, C reactive protein, and procalcitonin as early predictors of necrosis infection in acute necrotizing pancreatitis. Surgery 2003;133:257-262.

228. Brunkhorst FM, Eberhard OK, Brunkhorst R. Early identification of biliary pancreatitis with PCT. Am J Gastroenterol 1998;93:1191-1192.

229. Rau B, Frigerio I, Büchler M, Wegscheider K, Bassi C, Puolakkainen PA, et al. Evaluation of procalcitonin for predicting septic multiorgan failure and overall prognosis of secondary peritonitis. Arch Surg 2007;142:134-142.

230. Pindak D, Pechan J, Vavrecka A, Mifkovic A, Lutter I. The correlation of procalcitonin serum levels with the presence of biliary obstruction. Bratisl Lek Listy 2005; 10:373-374.

231. Rau B, Steinbach G, Gansauge F, Mayer M, Grünert A, Beger HG. The role of procalcitonin and interleukin-8 in the prediction of infected necrosis in acute pancreatitis. Gut 1997;41:832-840.

232. Martinot M, Hansmann Y, De Martino S, Lesens O, Coumaros G, Pencreach E, et al. La procalcitonine dans les pyelonephrites et les pneumopathies communautaires aigues de l'adulte. Presse Med 2001;30:1091-1096.

233. de Werra I, Jaccard C, Corradin SB, Chiolero R, Yersin B, Gallati H, et al. Cytokines, nitrite/nitrate, soluble tumor necrosis factor receptors, and procalcitonin concentrations: Comparisons in patients with septic shock, cardiogenic shock, and bacterial pneumonia. Crit Care Med 1997;25:607-613.

234. Brunkhorst FM, Clark AL, Forycki ZF, Anker SD. Pyrexia, procalcitonin, immune activation and survival in cardiogenic shock: the potential importance of bacterial translocation. International Journal of Cardiology 1999;72:3-10.

235. Geppert A, Steiner A, Delle-Karth G, Heinz G, Huber K. Usefulness of procalcitonin for diagnosing complicating sepsis in patients with cardiogenic shock. Intensive Care Med 2003;29:1384-1389.

236. Becker KL, Nylen ES, Arifi AA, Thompson KA, Snider RH, Alzeer A. Effekt of classic heatstroke on serum procalcitonin. Crit Care Med 1997;25:1362-1365.

237. Hausfater P, Hurtado M, Pease S, Juillien G, al. e. Is procalcitonin a marker of criticall illness in heatstroke? Intensive Care Med 2008;34:1377-1383.

238. Kettelhack C, Hohenberger P, Furchtbar S, Schulze G, Schlag PM. Procalcitonin als Marker der systemischen inflammatorischen Reaktion nach isolierter Extremitätenperfusion. Langenbecks Archiv Forumband 1998: 399-402.

239. Bihan H, Becker KL, Snider RH, Nylen E, Vittaz L, Lauret C, et al. Calcitonin precursor levels in human medullary thyroid carcinoma. Thyroid 2003;13(8):819-822.

240. Bolko P, Manuszewska-Jopek E, Michalek K, Wasko R, Jaskula M, Sowinski J. Efficacy of procalcitonin measurement in patients after total thyroidectomy due to medullary thyroid carcinoma. Archivum Immunologine et Therapiae Experimentalis 2003;51:415-419.

241. Ittner L, Born W, Rau B, Steinbach G, Fischer AJ. Circulating procalcitonin and cleavage products in septicemia compared with medullary thyroid carcinoma. Eur J Endocrinology 2002;147:727-731.

242. Matzaraki V, Alexandraki KI, Venetsanou K, Piperi C, Myrianthefs P, al. e. Evaluation of serum procalcito-

nin and interleukin-6 levels as markers of liver metastasis. Clinical Biochemistry 2007;40:336-342.

243. Remskar M, Horvat M, Hojker S, Noc M. Procalcitonin in patients with acute myocardial infarction. Wien Klin Wochenschr 2002;114:205-210.

244. Ciaccio M, Fugardi G, Titone L, Romano A, Giordano S, Bivona G, et al. Procalcitonin levels in plasma in oncohaematological patients with and without bacterial infections. Clin Chim Acta 2004;340:149-152.

245. Ammori BJ, Becker KL, Kite P, Snider RH, Nylen ES, White JC, et al. Calcitonin precursors: Early markers of gut barrier dysfunction in patients with acute pancreatitis. Pancreas 2003;27:239-243.

246. Elefsiniotis IS, Skounakis M, Vezali M, Pantazisa KD, Petrocheiloub A, Pirounakia M, et al. Clinical significance of serum procalcitonin levels in patients with acute or chronic liver disease. Eur J Gastroenterol Hepatol 2005;18:525-530.

247. Connert S, Stremmel W, Elsing C. Procalcitonin is a valid marker of infection in decompensated cirrhosis. Z Gastroenterol 2003;41:165-170.

248. Neely AN, Fowler LA, Kagan RJ, Warden GD. Procalcitonin in pediatric burn patients: an early indicator of sepsis? J Burn Care Rehabil 2004;25:76-80.

249. Dehne MG, Sabotzki A, Hoffmann A, Mühling J, Dietrich FE, Hempelmann G. Alterations of acute phase reaction and cytokine production in patients following sever burn injury. Burns 2002;28:535-542.

250. Sachse C, Machens HG, Felmerer G, Berger A, Henkel E. Procalcitonin as a marker for the early diagnosis of severe infection after thermal injury. J Burn Care Rehabil 1999;20:354-360.

251. Ulrich D, Noah EM, Pallua N. Plasma-Endotoxin, Procalcitonin, C-reaktives Protein und Organfunktionen bei Patienten mit schweren Brandverletzungen. Handchir Mikrochir Plast Chir 2001;33:262-266.

252. Carsin H, Assicot M, Feger F, Roy O, Pennacino I, Le Bever H, et al. Evolution and significance of circulating procalcitonin levels compared with IL-6, TNFα and endotoxin levels early after thermal injury. Burns 1997; 23:218-224.

253. von Heimburg D, Stieghorst W, Khorram-Sefat R, Pallua N. Procalcitonin – a sepsis parameter in severe burn injuries. Burns 1998;24:745-750.

254. Nylen E, O'Neill WJ, Jordan MH, Snider R, Moore CF, Lewis MS, et al. Serum Procalcitonin as an index of inhalation injury in burns. Horm Metab Res 1992;24: 439-442.

255. Becker KL, O'Neill WJ, Snider R, Nylen E, Moore CF, Jeng J, et al. Hyperprocalcitoninemia in inhalation burn injury: a response of the pulmonary neuroendocrine cell? Anat.Rec. 1993;236:136-138.

256. O'Neill WJ, Jordan MH, Lewis MS, Snider R, Moore CF, Becker KL. Serum calcitonin may be a marker for inhalation injury in burns. J Burn Care Rehabil 1992;13: 605-616.

257. Ueyama M, Maruyama I, Osame M. Marked increase in plasma interleukin-6 in burn patients. J Lab Clin Med 1992;120:693-698.

258. Yeh FL, Lin WL, Shen HD, Fang RH. Changes in levels of serum IL-8 in burned patients. Burns 1997;23(7-8):555-559.

259. Lavrentieva A, Kontakiotis T, Lazaridis L, Tsotolis N, Koumis J, Kyriazis G, et al. Inflammatory markers in patients with severe burn injury. What is the best indicator of sepsis? Burns 2006;33:189-194.

260. Chiesa C, Panero A, Rossi N, Stegagno M, De Giusti M, Osborn JF, et al. Reliability of procalcitonin concentrations for the diagnosis of sepsis in critically ill neonates. Clinical Infectious Diseases 1998;26:664-672.

261. Chiesa C, Pacifico L, Rossi N, Panero A, Matrunola M, Mancuso G. Procalcitonin as a marker of nosocomial infections in the neonatal intensive care unit. Intensive Care Med 2000;26:S175-S177.

262. Chiesa C, Pellegrini G, Pandero A, Osborn JF, Signore F, Assumma M, et al. C-reactive protein, interleukin-6, and procalcitonin in the immediate postnatal period: influence of illness severity, risk status, antenatal and perinatal complications, and infection. Clinical Chemistry 2003;49(1):60-68.

263. Nijsten MW, Olinga P, Hoekstra HJ. In vitro and in vivo stimulation of procalcitonin by TNFa and IL-6. Journal für Anästhesie und Intensivtherapie 2001;2:58-60.

264. Hambach L, Eder M, Dammann E, Schrauder A, Sykora KW, Dieterich C, et al. Diagnostic value of procalcitonin serum levels in comparison with C-reactive protein in allogeneic stem cell transplantation. Haematologica 2002;87:643-651.

265. Kuse ER, Jaeger K. Procalcitonin increase after anti-CD3 monoclonal antibody therapy does not indicate infectious disease. Transpl Int 2001;14:55.

266. Sabat R, Höflich C, Döcke WD, Oppert M, Kern F, Windrich B, et al. Massive elevation of procalcitonin plasma levels in the absence of infection in kidney transplant patients treated with pan-T-cell antibodies. Intensive Care Med 2001;27:987-991.

267. Dornbusch HJ, Strenger V, Kerbl R, Lackner H, Schwinger W, Sovinz P, et al. Procalcitonin and C-reactive protein do not discriminate between febrile reaction to anti-T-lymphocyte antibodies and Gram-negative sepsis. Bone Marrow Transplantation 2003;32:941-945.

268. Madershahian N, Wittwer T, Franke UFW, Wippermann J, Strauch J, Groetzner J, et al. Effect of induction

therapy on kinetic on procalcitonin following uncomplicated heart transplantation. J Card Surg 2007;22:199-202.

269. Sarbinowski R, Arvidsson S, Tylman M, Öresland T, Bengtsson A. Plasma concentrations of procalcitonin and systemic inflammatory response syndrome after colorectal surgery. Acta Anaestehesiol Scand 2005;49: 191-196.

270. Mokart D, Merlin M, Sannini A, Brun JP, Delpero JP, Houvenaeghel G, et al. Procalcitonin, interleukin 6 and ystemic inflammatory response syndrome (SIRS): early markers of postoperative sepsis after major surgery. Br J Anaesth 2005;94:767-773.

271. Dörge H, Schöndube FA, Dörge P, Seipelt R, Voss M, Messmer BJ. Procalcitonin is a valuable prognostic marker in cardiac surgery but not specific for infection. Thorac Cardiov Surg 2003;51:322-326.

272. Molter GP, Soltesz S, Kottke R, Wilhelm W, Biedler A, Silomon M. Procalcitonin plasma concentrations and systemic inflammatory response following different types of surgery. Anaesthesist 2003;52:210-217.

273. Sauerland S, Hensler T, Bouillon B, Rixen D, Raum MR, Adermahr J, et al. Plasma levels of procalcitonin and neopterin in multiple trauma patients with or without brain injury. Journal of Neurotrauma 203;20:953-960.

274. Mimoz O, Benoist JF, Edouard AR, Assicot M, Bohoun C, Samii K. Procalcitonin and C-reactive protein during the early posttraumatic systemic inflammatory response syndrome. Intensive Care Med 1998;24: 185-188.

275. Reith HB, Mittelkötter U, Debus ES, Kussner C, Thiede A. Procalcitonin in early detection of postoperative complications. Dig Surg 1998;15:260-265.

276. Kuse ER, Langefeld I, Jaeger K, Kulpmann WR. Procalcitonin in fever of unknown origin after liver transplantation: a variable to differentiate acute rejection from infection. Crit Care Med 2000;28:555-559.

277. Fazakas J, Gondos T, Varga M, Sarvary E, Horovitz P, Pemer F. Analysis of systemic and regional procalcitonin serum levels during liver transplantation. Transplant International 2003;16(7):465-470.

278. Kunz D. Diagnostic relevance of procalcitonin, IL-6 and cellular immune status in the early phase after liver transplantation. Transplant Proc 1998;30:2398-2399.

279. Ito S, Sato N, Kojika M, Yaegashi Y, Suzuki Y, Suzuki K, et al. Serum procalcitonin levels are elevated in esophageal cancer patients with postoperative infectious complications. Eur Surg Res 2005;37:22-28.

280. Meisner M, Tschaikowsky K, Hutzler A, Schmidt J, Harig F, von der Emde J. Postoperative plasma concentrations of procalcitonin and C-reactive protein after cardiothoracic surgery with and without extracorporeal circulation. British Journal of Anaesthesia 1998;80 (suppl. 1):79.

281. Guz G, Colak B. Procalcitonin and conventional markers of inflammation in peritoneal dialysis patients and peritonitis. Peritoneal Dialysis International 2006; 26:240-248.

282. Chromik AM, Endter F, Uhl W, Thiede A, Reith HB, Mittelkötter U. Pre-emptive antibiotic treatment vs "standard" treatment in patients with elevated serum procalcitonin levels after elective colorectal surgery: a prospective randomised pilot study. Langenbecks Arch Surg 2006;391(3):187-194.

283. Loebe M, Lociewski S, Brunkhorst FM, Harke C, Hetzer R. Procalcitonin in patients undergoing cardiopulmonary bypass in open heart surgery- first results of the procalcitonin in heart surgery study (ProHearts). Intensive Care Med 2000;26 (S2):193-198.

284. Aouifi A, Piriou V, Blanc P, Bouvier H, Bastien O, Chiari P, et al. Effect of cardiopulmonary bypass on serum procalcitonin and C-reactive protein concentrations. Br J Anaesth 1999;83:602-607.

285. Yasmin D, Bulut G, Yildiz M. Can procalcitonin be used for the diagnosis and follow-up of postoperative complications after fracture surgery? Acta Orthop Traumatol Turc 2006;40(1):15-21.

286. Aouifi A, Piriou V, Bastien, Blanc P, Bouvier H, Evans R, et al. Usefulness of procalcitonin for diagnosis of infection in cardiac surgical patients. Crit Care Med 2000;28(9):3171-3176.

287. Boeken U, Feindt P, Micek M, Petzold T, Schulte HD, Gams E. Procalcitonin (PCT) in cardiac surgery: diagnostic value in systemic inflammatory resonse syndrome (SIRS), sepsis and after heart transplantation (HTX). Cardiovascular Surgery 2000;8(7):550-554.

288. Arkader R, Troster EJ, Abellan DM, Lopez MR, Raiz R, Carciallo JA, et al. Procalcitonin and C-reactive protein kinetics in postoperative pediatric cardiac surgical patients. J Cardiothoracic and Vascular Anaesthesia 2004;18(2):160-165.

289. Beghetti M, Rimensberger PC, Kalangos A, Habre W, Gervaix A. Kinetics of procalcitonin, interleukin-6 and C-reactive protein after cardiopulmonary-bypass in children. Cardiol Young 2003;13:161-167.

290. Celebi S, Koner O, Menda F, Balci H, Hatemi A, Korkut K, et al. Procalcitonin kinetics in pediatric patients with systemic inflammatory response after open heart surgery. Intensive Care Med 2006;DOI 10.1007/ s00134-006-0180-z.

291. Baykut D, Schulte-Herbrüggen J, Krian A. The value of procalcitonin as an infection marker in cardiac surgery. Eur J Med Res 2000;5:530-536.

292. Bach F, Grundmann U, Bauer M, Buchinger H, Soltesz S, Graeter T, et al. Modulation of the inflammatory response to cardiopulmonary bypass by dopexamine and epidural anesthesia. Acta Anaestehsiol Scand 2002; 46:1227-1235.

293. Falcoz PE, Laluc F, Toubin MM, Puyraveau M, Clement F, Mercier M, et al. Usefulness of procalcitonin in the early detection of infection after thoracic surgery. Eur J Cardiothorac Surg 2005;27:1074-1078.

294. Kornberg A, Grube T, Wagner T, Voigt R, Homman M, Schotte U, et al. Differentiated therapy with prostaglandin E1 (Alprostadil) after orthotopic liver transplantation: the usefulness of procalcitonin (PCT) and hepatic artery resistive index (RI) for the evaluation of early graft function and clinical course. Clin Chem Lab Med 2000; 38:1177-1180.

295. Staehler M, Hammer C, Meiser B, Reichart B. Procalcitonin: a new marker for differential diagnosis of acute rejection and bacterial infection in heart transplantation. Transplantation proceedings 1997;29:584-585.

296. Hammer S, Meisner F, Dirschedl P, Höbel G, Fraunberger P, Meiser B, et al. Procalcitonin: a new marker for diagnosis of acute rejection and bacterial infection in patients after heart and lung transplantation. Transpl Immunol 1998;6:235-241.

297. Staehler M, Überfuhr P, Reichart B, Hammer C. Differentialdiagnostik der Abstossungsreaktion und Infektion bei herztransplantierten Patienten: neue Wege mit Zytokinen und Procalcitonin als Marker. Transplantationsmedizin 1997;9:44-50.

298. Potapov EV, Wagner DF, Loebe M, Ivanitskaia EA, Müller C, Sodian R, et al. Elevated donor cardiac troponin T and procalcitonin indicate two independent mechanisms of early graft failure after heart transplantation. Internat J Cardiology 2003;92:163-167.

299. Langefeld I, Schulzeck P, Schlitt HJ, Oldhafer K, Jaeger K, Kruse E-R. Procalcitonin (PCT) zur Differenzierung zwischen Infektion und Abstossung beim Transplantierten mit FUO. AINS 1997;32:10.7.

300. Striz I, Jaresova M, Lacha J, Sedlacek J, Vitko S. MRP 8/14 and Procalcitonin serum levels in organ transplantations. Annals of Transplantation 2001;6(2):6-9.

301. Herget-Rosenthal S, Klein T, Marggraf G, Hirsch T, Jakob HG, Philipp T, et al. Modulation and source of procalcitonin in reduced renal function and renal replacement therapy. Scandinavian Journal of Immunology 2005;61:180-186.

302. Steinbach G, Bölke E, Grünert A, Orth K, Störck M. Procalcitonin in patients with acute and chronic renal insufficiencyc. Wien Klin Wochenschr 2004;116(24): 849-853.

303. Sitter T, Schmidt M, Schneider S, Schiffl H. Differential diagnosis of bacterial infection and inflammatory response in kidney disease using procalcitonin. J Nephrol 2002;15:297-301.

304. Chauveau P, Level C, Lasseur C, Bonarek H, al. e. C-reactive protein and procalcitonin as markers of mortality in hemodialysis patients: a 2-year prospective study. Journal of Renal Nutrition 2003;13(2):137-143.

305. Dahaba AA, Rehak PH, List WF. Procalcitonin and C-reactive protein plasma concentrations in nonseptic uremic patients undergoing hemodialysis. Intensive Care Med 2003;29:579-583.

306. Schmidt M, Burchardi C, Sitter T, Held E, Schiffl H. Procalcitonin in patients undergoing chronic hemodialysis. Nephron 2000;84:187-188.

307. Lorton F, Veinberg F, Ielsch D, Deschênes G, Bensman A, Ulinski T. Procalcitonin serum levels in children undergoing chronic haemodialysis. Pediatr Nephrol 2006;DOI 10.1007/s00467-006-0304-2.

308. Meisner M, Hüttemann E, Lohs T, Kasakov L, Reinhart K. Plasma concentrations and clearance of procalcitonin during continuous veno-venous hemofiltration in septic patients. Shock 2001;15:171-175.

309. Dahaba AA, Elawady GA, Rehak.P.H., List WF. Procalcitonin and proinflammatory cytokine clearance during continuous venovenous haemofiltrations in septic patients. Anaesth Intensive Care 2002;30:269-274.

310. Meisner M, Hüttemann E, Lohs T, Kasakov L, Reinhart K. Elimination of procalcitonin and plasma concentrations during continuous veno-venous haemodiafiltration in septic patients. Eur J Anaesthesiol 2000;17: 665-671.

311. Herget-Rosenthal S, Marggraf G, Pietruck F, Hüsing J, Strupat M, Philipp T, et al. Procalcitonin for acurate detection of infection in haemodialysis. Nephrol Dial Transplant 2001;16:975-979.

312. Becker KL, Gazdar AF, Carney DN, Snider RH, Moore CF, Silva OL. Calcitonin secretion by continuous cultures of small cell carcinoma of the lung: Incidence and immunoheterogeniety studies. Cancer Lett. 1983;18: 179-185.

313. Penel N, Fournier C, Degardin M, Kouto H, Guyen MN. Fievre et tumeur solide: valeur diagnostique de la procalcitonine et de la proteine C reactive. Rev Med Interne 2001;22:706-714.

314. Ilhan N, Ilhan N, Ilhan Y, Akbulut H, Kücüksu M. C-reactive protein, procalcitonin, interleukin-6, vascular endothelial growth factor and oxidative metabolites in diagnosis of infection and staging in patients with gastric cancer. World J Gastroenterol 2004;10(8):1115-1120.

315. Fleischhack G, Kambeck I, Cipic D, Hasan C, Bode U. Procalcitonin in paediatric cancer patients: its diagnostic relevance is superior to that of C-reactive protein, interleukin 6, interleukin 8, soluble interleukin 2 receptor and soluble tumor necrosis factor receptor II. British Journal of Haematology 2000;111:1093-1102.

316. Fleischhack G, Cipic D, Juettner J, Hasan C, Bode U. Procalcitonin – A sensitive inflammation marker of febrile episodes in neutropenic children with cancer. Intensive Care Med 2000;26:S202-S211.

317. von Lilienfeld-Toal M, Dietrich MP, Glasmacher A, Lehmann L, Breig P, Hahn C, et al. Markers of bacteremia in febrile neutropenic patients with hematologic malignancies: procalcitonin and IL-6 are more reliable than CRP. Eur J Clin Microbiol Infect Dis 2004;23:539-544.

318. Secmeer G, Devrim I, Kara A, Ceyhan M, et al. Role of procalcitonin and CRP in differentiating a stable from a deteriorating clincal course in pediatric febrile neutropenia. J Pediatr Hematol Oncol 2007;29:107-111.

319. Sauer M, Tiede K, Fuchs D, Gruhn B, Berger D, Zintl F. Procalcitonin, C-reactive protein, and endotoxin after bone marrow transplantation: identification of children at high risk of morbidity and mortality from sepsis. Bone Marrow Transplantation 2003;31:1137-1142.

320. Giamarellou H, Giamarellos-Bourboulis EJ, Repoussis P, Galani L, Anagnostopoulos N, Grecka P, et al. Potential use of procalcitonin as a diagnostic criterion in febrile neutropenia: experience from a multicentre study. Clin Microbiol Infect 2004;10:628-633.

321. Fleischhack G, Kambeck I, Cipic D, Hasan C, Bode U. Reply to De Bont et al. Br J Hematol 2001;114:490-491.

322. Engel A, Steinbach G, Kern P, Kern WV. Diagnostic value of procalcitonin serum levels in neutropenic patients with fever: comparison with IL-8. Scand J Infect Dis 1999;31:185-189.

323. Bernard L, Ferriere F, Casassus P, Malas F, Leveque S, Guillevin L, et al. Procalcitonin as an early marker of bacterial infection in severly neutropenic febrile adults. Clin Infect Dis 1998;27:914-915.

324. Schüttrumpf S, Binder L, Hagemann T, Berkovic D, Trümper L, Binder C. Procalcitonin: a useful discriminator between febrile conditions of different origin in hemato-oncological patients? Ann Hematol 2003;82:98-103.

325. Svaldi M, Hirber J, Lanthaler AI, Mayr O, Faes S, Peer E, et al. Procalcitonin-reduced sensitivity and specificity in heavily leucopenic and immunosuppressed patients. Br J Haematol 2001;115:53-57.

326. de Bont ESJM, Kamps W, Vellenga E, Swaanenburg J. Procalcitonin: a diagnostic marker of bacterial infection in neutropenic cancer patients with fever? Infection 2000;28:398-400.

327. Kitanovski L, Jazbec J, Hojker S, Gubina M, Derganc M. Diagnostic accuracy of procalcitonin and interleukin-6 values for predicting bacteremia and clinical sepsis in febrile neutropenic children with cancer. Eur J Clin Microbiol Infect Dis 2006;25:413-415.

328. Zintl F, Sauer M, Fuchs D, Hermann J, Reinhart K. High serum procalcitonin (PCT) concentrations in children and adults after hemopoietic stemm cell transplantation(HSCT) – an indictor for poor prognosis in severe infections. Blood, suppl.1 1996;88:266.

329. Blijlevens NMA, Donnelly JP, Meis FGM, De Keizer MH, De Pauw BE. Procalcitonin does not discriminate infection from inflammation after allogeneic bone marrow transplantation. Clinical and Diagnostic Laboratory Immunology 2000;7:889-892.

330. Turner D, Hammerman C, Rudensky B, Schlesinger Y, Goia C, Schimmel MS. Procalcitonin in preterm infants during the first few days of life: introducing an age related nomogram. Arch Dis Chiold Fetal Neonatal 2006;9:F283-286.

331. Lopez Sastre JB, Solis DP, Serradilla VR, Colomer BF, Cotallo GDC, al. e. Evaluation of procalcitonin for diagnosis of neonatal sepsis of vertical transmission. BMC Pediatrics 2007;7:1-9.

332. Stocker M, Fontana M, el Helou S, Wegscheider K, Berger TM. Effect of procalcitonin-guided decision making on duration of antibiotic therapy in suspected neonatal early-onset sepsis: Prospective randomized intervention trial. Neonatology 2010;97:165-174.

333. Carrol ED, Newland P, Riordan FAI, Thomson APJ, Curtis N, Hart CA. Procalcitonin as a diagnostic marker of meningococcal disease in children presenting with fever and a rash. Arch Dis Child 2002;86:282-285.

334. Rey C, Los Arcos M, Concha A, Medina A, Prieto S, Martinez P, et al. Procalcitonin and C-reactive protein as markers of systemic inflammatory response syndrome severity in critically ill patients. Intensive Care Med 2007; DOI.

335. Herd D. In children under age three does procalcitonin help exclude serious bacterial infection in fever without focus? Arch Dis Child 2007;92:362-368.

336. Bohuon C, Assicot M, Raymond J, Gendrel D. Procalcitonin, a marker of bacterial meningitis in children in childhood. Bull Acad Natl Med 1998;182:1469-1475.

337. Liu CF, Cai XX, Wei X. Serum procalcitonin levels in children with bacterial or viral meningitis. China 2006;8(1):17-20.

338. Bienvenu J, Monneret G, Isaac G, Bienvenu F, Putet G, Floret G. Procalcitonin in bacterial and viral infec-

tions in premature infants and neonates. Schock 1997; suppl. 1.

339. Gendrel D, Assicot M, Raymond J, Moulin F, Francoul C, Badoual J, et al. Procalcitonin as a marker for the early diagnosis of neonatal infection. J Pediatrics 1996; 128:570-573.

340. Saez-Llorens X, McCraecken GHJ. Perinatal bacterial disease. In. Felgin, R.D., Cherry, J.D. eds. Textbook of pediatric infectious diseases. Philadelphia: WB Saunders 1998:892-926.

341. Janota J, Stranak Z, Belohlavkova S, Mudra K, Simak J. Postnatal increase of procalcitonin in premature newborns is enhanced by chorioamnionitis and neonatal sepsis. European Journal of Clinical Investigation 2001; 31:978-983.

342. Kordek A, Giedrys-Kalemba S, Pawlus B, Podraza W, Czajka R. Umbilical cord blood serum procalcitonin concentration in the diagnosis of early neonatal infection. Journal of Perinatology 2003;23:148-153.

343. Köksal N, Harmanci R, Cetinkaya M, Hacimustafaoglu M. Role of procalcitonin and CRP in diagnosis and follow-up of neonatal sepsis. The Turkish Journal of Pediatrics 2007;49:21-29.

344. Chiesa C, Pacifico L, Mancuso G, Panero A. Procalcitonin in pediatrics: overview and challenge. Infection 1998;26:238-241.

345. Mariscalco MM. Is plasma procalcitonin ready for prime time in the pediatric intensive care unit? Pediatr Crit Care Med 2003;4(1):118-119.

346. Kunz D, Kohse KP. Entzündungsdiagnostik in der Pädiatrie. J Lab Med 2002;26:335-340.

347. Leclerc F, Herbomez MD. Procalcitonin in the pediatric ICU. Archives de Pediatre 2004;11:587-589.

348. van Rossum AMC, Wulkan RW, Oudesluys-Murphy AM. Procalcitonin as an early marker of infection in neonates and children. Lancet Infect Dis 2004; 4:620-630.

349. Hsiao AL, Baker MD. Fever in the new millennium: a review of recent studies of markers of serious bacterial infections in febrile children. Curr Opin Pediatr 2005; 17:56-61.

350. Kordek A, Torbe A, Czajka R. Maternal venous procalcitonin levels do not correlate with umbilical cord and venous blood concentrations in the neonate. J Pernat Med 2006;34:462-465.

351. Vazzalwar R, Pina-Rodrigues E, Puppala BL, Angst DB, Schweig L. Procalcitonin as a screening test for late-onset sepsis in preterm very low birth weight infants. Journal of Perinatology 2005;1:1-6.

352. Turner D, Hammermann C, Rudensky B, Schlesinger Y, Schlesinger M, Schimmel S. The role of procalcitonin as a predictor of nosocomial sepsis in preterm infants. Acta Paediatrica 2006;95:1571-1576.

353. Guibourdenche J, Bedu A, Petzold L, Marchand M, Mariani-Kurdijan P, Hurtaud-Roux MF, et al. Biochemical markers of neonatal sepsis: value of procalcitonin in the emergency setting. Ann Clin Biochem 2002;39: 130-135.

354. Resch B, Gusenleitner W, Müller WD. Procalcitonin and Interleukin-6 in the diagnosis of early-onset sepsis of the neonate. Acta Paediatr 2003;92:243-245.

355. Kocabas E, Sarikcioglu A, Aksary N, Seydaoglu G, Seyhun Y, Yaman A. Role of procalcitonin, C-reactive protein, interleukin-6, interleukin-8 and tumor necrosis factor alpha in the diagnosis of neonatal sepsis. The Turkish Journal of Pediatrics 2007;(49):7-20.

356. Hochreiter M, Köhler T. et al. Antibiotikatherapie bei operativen Intensivpatienten. Anaesthesist 2008;57: 571-577.

357. Krüger S, Ewig S, Marre R et al. Procalcitonin predicts patients at low risk of death from community-acquired pneumonia across all CRB-65 classes. Eur Respir J 2008;31:349-355.

358. Franzin L, Cabodi D. Legionella Pneumonia and Serum Procalcitonin. Current Microbiology 2005;50:43-46.

359. Maisel A, Anker SD, et al. Biomarkers in the Assessment of Congestive Heart Failure. Submitted 2009.

360. Morath C, Sis J, Haensch MG, Zeier M, Andrassay K, Schwenger V. Procalcitonin as marker of infection in patients with Goodpasture´s syndrome is misleading. Nephrol Dial Transplant 2007;22:2701-2704.

361. Fries M, Kunz D, Gressner AM, Roissant R, Kuhlen R. Procalcitonin serum levels after out-of-hospital cardiac arrest. Resuscitation 2003;59:105-109.

362. Oppert M, Reinicke A, Müller C, Barckow D, Frei U, Eckard KU. Elevations in procalcitonin but not C-reactive protein are associated with pneumonia after cardiopulmonary resuscitation. Resuscitation 2002;53:167-170.

363. Spahr L, Morard I, Hadengue A, Vadas L, Pugin J. Procalcitonin is not an accurate marker of spontaneous bacterial peritonitis in patients with cirrhosis. Hepato-Gastroenterology 2001;48:502-505.

364. Amour J, Birenbaum A, Langeron O, et al. Influence of renal dysfunction on the accuracy of procalcitonin for the diagnosis of postoperative infection after vascular surgery. Crit Care Med 2008;36:1147-1154.

365. Sexton PM, Christopoulos G, Christopoulos A, Nylen ES, Snider RH, Becker KL. Procalcitonin has bioactivity at calcitonin receptor family compexes: Potential mediator implications in sepsis. Crit Care Med 2008; 36:1637-1640.

366. Algeciras-Schimnich A, Preissner CM, Theobald JP, Finseth MS, Grebe SK. Procalcitonin: a marker for the diagnosis and follow-up of patients with medullary thyroid carcinoma. J Clin Endocrinol Metab 2009; 94:861-868.

367. Endo S, Aikawa N, Fujishima S, Sekine I et al. Usefulness of procalcitonin serum level for the discrimination of sepsis from severe sepsis: a multicenter prospective study. J Infect Chemother 2008; 14:244-249.

368. Maniaci V, Dauber A, Weiss S, Nylen E, Becker KL, Bachur R. Procalcitonin in young febrile infants for the detection of serious bacterial infections. Pediatrics 2008; 122:701-10.

369. Schroeder S, Hochreiter M, Koehler T, Schweiger AM, Bein B, Keck FS, von Spiegel T. Procalcitonin (PCT)-guided algorithm reduces length of antibiotic treatment in surgical intensive care patients with severe sepsis: result of a prospective randomized study. Langbecks Arch Surg 2009;394:221-226.

370. Viallon et al. Can emergency physicians identify a high mortality subgroup of patients with sepsis: role of procalctionin. Eur J Emergency Medicine 2008;15:26-33.

371. Stolz D, Smyrnios N, Eggimann P, Pargger H, Thakkar N, Siegemund M, Marsch S, Rakic J, Mueller B, Tamm M. Procalcitonin for reduced antibiotic exposure in ventilator associated pneumonia – a randomized study. Eur Respir J 2009;34(6):1364-1375.

372. O'Grady NP, Barie PS, Barlett JG, Bleck T et al. Guidelines for evaluation of new fever in critically ill adult patients: 2008 update from the American College of Critical Care Medicine and the Infectious Diseases Society of America. Crit Care Med 2008; 36:1330-1349.

373. Hausfater P, Juillien G, Madonna-Py B et al. Serum procalcitonin measurement as diagnostic and prognostic marker in febrile adult patients presenting to the emergency department. Crital Care 2007; 11:R60.

374. Conti G, Amore A, Chiesa M, Mancuso D et al. Procalcitonin as a marker of micro-inflammation in hemodialysis. J Nephrol 2005; 18:282-288.

375. Schützle H, Forster J, Superti-Furga A, Berner R. Is serum procalcitonin a reliable diagnostic marker in children with acute respiratory tract infection? A retrospective analysis. Eur J Pediatr 2009;168:1117-1124.

376. Nseir S, Cavestri B, Di Pompeo C et al. Factors predicting bacterial involvement in severe acute exacerbations of chronic obstructive pulmonary disease. Respiration 2008; 76:253-260.

377. Schuetz P, Mueller B, Trampuz A. Serum procalcitonin for discriminatino of blood contaminatino from boodstream infection due to coagulase-negative staphylococci. Infection 2007; 35: 352-355.

378. Sakr Y, Sponholz C, Tuche F, Brunkhorst F, Reinhart K. The role of procalcitonin in febrile neutropenic patients: Review of the literature. Infection 2008; 36:396-407.

379. Sakr Y, Burgett U, Nacul FE, Reinhart K, Brunkhorst F. Lipopolysaccharide binding protein in a surgical intensive care unit: a marker of sepsis? Crit Care Med 2008; 36:2014-2022.

380. Galetto-Lacour A, Zamora SA, Gervaix A. A score identifying serious bacterial infections in children with fever without source. Pediatric Infect Dis J 2008; 27: 654-656.

381. Mills GD, Lala HM, Oehley MR, Craig AM et al. Elevated procalcitonin as a diagnostic marker in meningococcal disease. Eur J Clin Microbiol Infect Dis 2006; 25: 501-509.

382. Casado-Flores J, Blanco-Quiros A, Montserrat, Asensio J, Fernandez C. Prognostic utility of the semiquantitative procalcitonin test, neutrophil count and C-reactive protein in meningococcal infection in children. Eur J Pediatr. 2006; 165:26-29.

383. Ramirez P, Sequential measurements of procalcitonin levels in diagnosing ventilator-associated pneumonia. Eur Respir J. 2008; 31:356-362.

384. Linscheid P, Seboek D, Nylen ES, Langer I, Schlatter M, Keller U, Becker KL, Müller B. In vitro and in vivo calcitonin-I gene expression in parenchymal cells: a novel product of human adipose tissue. Endocrinology 2003; 144:5578-5584.

385. Schuetz P, Christ-Crain M, Thomann R, Falconnier C et al. Effect of procalcitonin-based guidelines vs standard guidelines on antibiotic use in lower respiratory tract infections. JAMA 2009;302:1059-1066.

386. Joram N, Boscher C, Denizot S, Loubersac V, Winer N, Roze JC, Gras-Le Gruen C. Umbilical cord blood procalcitonin and C-reactive protein concentrations as marker for early diagnosis of very early onset neonatal infection. Arch Dis Child Fetal Neonatal 2006;91:F65-66.

387. Isidor B, Cailiaux G, Gilquin V, Loubersac V, Caillon J, Roze JC, Gras-Le Gruen C. The use of procalcitonin in the diagnosis of late-onset infection in neonatal intensive care unit patients. Scand J Infect Dis 2007;39: 1063-1066.

388. Hatzistilianou M, Tekleity A, Athanassiadou F, DeLutils MA, Conti P, Catrin D. Serum procalcitonin responses in infection of children with secondary immunodeficiency. Clin Invest Med 2007;30:E75-85.

389. Bouadma L, Luyt CE, Tubach F, Cracco C, Alvarez A, Schwebel C, Schortgen F, Lasocki S et al. Use of Procalcitonin to shorten ICU patients´ exposure to anti-

biotics – the randomized controlled PRORATA trial. Lancet 2010;375(9713):463-474.

390. Schüttrumpf S, Binder L, Hagemann T, Berkovic D, Trümper L, Binder C. Utility of procalcitonin concentration in the evaluation of patients with malignant diseases and elevated C-reactive protein plasma concentrations. Clin Infect Dis 2006;43:468-473.

Index

A

absolute values ... 13
airway infections ... 57
allergic diseases ... 74
amino acid sequence ... 9, 33
amniorrhexis, premature ... 96
antibiotic therapy
  duration ... 55
  effectiveness ... 55
  frequency of prescription ... 52
  in airway infections ... 57
  in exacerbation of COPD ... 59
  in patients in intensive care ... 62
  indication ... 15, 25
  individual, patient-adapted (IPAT) ... 52
  monitoring ... 15, 25
  PCT-controlled ... 32, 54
  reasons for prescription ... 31
  studies ... 57
anti-lymphocyte globulins ... 81
anti-neutrophil antibody-positive vasculitis ... 73
appendicitis ... 104
aspergillus infections ... 72
autoimmune diseases ... 40, 41, 73, 81

B

bacteremia ... 67
bacterial infections ... 10
  differential diagnosis ... 19, 40
  in children ... 101
  therapy ... 17
biochemical properties ... 16
biochemistry ... 33
biological effects ... 36
burns ... 81

C

candida infections ... 72
cardiogenic shock ... 80
C-cell carcinoma of the thyroid gland ... 87
cerebral external ventricle drainages (EVD) ... 104
chemotherapy ... 88
children
  diagnoses ... 97
  infections ... 40
  measuring PCT levels ... 92
cholecystitis ... 104
cirrhosis of the liver ... 80
community-acquired pneumonia (CAP)
  antibiotic therapy ... 58, 60
CRP ... 17, 41, 42, 47, 48

D

diagnostic use ... 10, 17
dialysis ... 87

E

elderly ... 81
elevated values
  interpretation ... 21
elimination ... 35
  renal ... 86
emergency room ... 27
endocarditis, bacterial ... 68
endotoxin ... 50
exacerbation of COPD ... 59
examples of use ... 29, 32
extracorporal circulation ... 83

F

false-positive levels ... 81
fever in children ... 77
frequency of measurements ... 103
fungal diseases ... 72

G

genetics ... 34
golden hours of early therapy ... 46
Goodpasture's Syndrome ... 73

H

half-life ... 39
heart surgery ... 83
heat shock ... 81
hematological/oncological illnesses ... 88
hemodiafiltration ... 87
hemodialysis ... 80
hemofiltration ... 80, 87
hepatitis, viral ... 80
HLA-DR ... 51

I

IL-6 ... 17, 41, 50
induction ... 35
  comparison with other markers ... 84
infants ... 97
infections, severe ... 42
intensive care unit ... 26, 40
  antibiotic therapy ... 62
interpretation ... 19, 46
  for IPAT ... 54
IPAT ... 52, 105
  goals and requirements ... 53
  in CAP ... 60
  interpretation of PCT ... 54

K

Kawasaki Syndrome ... 73
kinetics ... 15

L

laboratory chemistry ...39
lactate ...17
LBP ...51
leukemia ...90
leukopenia ...90
local infections ...42
low birth weight ...97
lymphomas ...90

M

MBL ...51
measurement in the urine ...86
medullary carcinoma of the thyroid gland ...87
meningitis, acute ...40, 69
  serum levels of PCT ...70
meningococcal infection ...100
methods of PCT level measurement ...39
MIF ...51
MR-proADM ...51
MR-proANP ...51
multiple organ dysfunction ...80

N

neopterin ...41
neutropenia ...89, 90
newborns ...81
non-bacterially induced formation ...79
non-inflammatory diseases ...81
normal range ...9, 39
  interpretation ...20

O

operations ...80
organ transplantation ...41
outpatient cases ...30
  antibiotic therapy ...30
  evaluation of PCT ...30

P

pancreatitis ...40, 74, 80, 104
PARTI study ...60
pathophysiology ...33
pediatric emergencies ...42
perfusion disorders ...80
peritonitis
  PCT serum concentration ...65
pneumonia ...40
  community-acquired ...60, 65
  diagnosis ...20, 65, 104
  nosocomial ...61, 65
  PCT serum concentration ...65
  ventilator-associated ...61
polytrauma ...83
preanalytical factors ...39
premature births ...97
pre-test probability ...14
ProCAP study ...60
ProCOLD study ...59
prognostic significance ...12
  in sepsis and severe bacterial infections ...23
progression ...23
  evaluation ...14
  in sepsis and severe bacterial infections ...23
  towards severe sepsis ...43
progression evaluation ...17, 45
proinflammatory cytokines ...81
properties ...10
PRORATA trial ...64
ProResp study ...58
prosthesis, infected ...104
pyelonephritis ...76

Q

quick test (PCT-Q) ...103

R

rejection reaction ...41
renal insufficiency ...80, 86
resuscitation ...80
risk evaluation ...44

S

sensitivity ...17
  comparison with other markers ...49
  differentiation of SIRS and sepsis ...43
sepsis ...10, 40, 42
  diagnosis ...17
  differential diagnosis ...19
  evaluation of severity ...22
  in infants and toddlers ...97
  monitoring ...22
  mortality ...11
  newborn ~ ...93
  progression ...12
  serum and plasma concentrations of PCT ...43
  severe ...17
  therapy ...17
septic shock
  diagnosis ...17
severity of disease ...10
SOFA score ...11
solid tumors ...90
special indications ...65
specificity ...12, 17
  comparison with other markers ...49
  differentiation of SIRS and sepsis ...43
stability ...15, 39
sTREM-1 ...51
surgery ...81
systemic inflammatory reactions ...9
  evaluation of severity ...22
Systemic Inflammatory Response Syndrome (SIRS) ...40, 42
  mortality ...11
  serum and plasma concentrations of PCT ...43
systemic lupus erythematosis ...74

T

therapeutic consequences 103
toddlers 97
transplantation 80, 85
  bone marrow 91
  heart 83, 85
  hematopoetic stem cells 91
  kidney 40, 83, 85
  liver 83, 85
trauma 80, 81
tumor diseases 81, 87

U

umbilical cord blood 96
urinary tract infections 76, 102

V

vesicourethral reflux 76, 102
viral infections 41
  differential diagnosis 71
  in children 101

W

Wegener's Disease 73